Stepping Into The Dark...

Stepping Into The Dark...

David Lucas

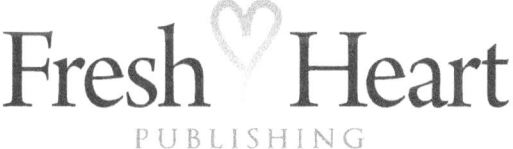

PUBLISHING

First published in Great Britain in 2010 by
FRESH HEART PUBLISHING
a division of Fresh Heart
PO Box 225, Chester le Street, DH3 9BQ, UK
www.freshheartpublishing.co.uk

© Fresh Heart Publishing 2010

The moral right of David Lucas to be identified as the author of this work has been asserted in accordance with the Copyright, Designs and Patents Act 1988.

All rights reserved. No part of this publication may be reproduced, stored in a retrieval system, or transmitted, in any form or by any means, electronic, mechanical, photocopying, recording or otherwise, without the prior permission of the publisher. Nor may this publication be circulated in any form of binding or cover other than that in which it is published and without a similar condition being imposed on the subsequent purchaser.

A CIP catalogue record for this book is available from the British Library

ISBN: 978 1 906619 17 6

Fresh Heart Life Changer series editor: Sylvie Donna
Cover design by Fresh Heart Publishing
Cover photograph by Shirley Hough
Designed and typeset by Fresh Heart Publishing
Set in Eras (medium, demi and light ITC) and Bradley Hand ITC

Printed and bound in Great Britain by Lightning Source UK Ltd
Printed and bound in the USA by Lightning Source Inc

Disclaimer

While the comments, advice and information contained in this book are believed to be accurate and true at the time of going to press, neither the author nor the publisher can accept any legal responsibility for loss, damage or injury occasioned to any person acting or refraining from action as a result of information contained herein. Advice is intended as a guideline only.

Dedication

This is for Tessa. She was a grand old lady of 16 but still she left us far too soon.

She was the most stubborn, wilful and sullen bitch you could ever come across. She always went her own way and seldom did as she was told. But she filled our home with love, joy and atmosphere.

And now she's gone. We miss her dreadfully. She changed our world and led us through the hardest of times. She never once let us down.

Sleep tight, old girl.

Contents

Foreword	A glimpse into what matters	ix
Introduction	My blockbuster?	1
Chapter 1	Déjà vu	4
Chapter 2	Consultation	9
Chapter 3	An image makeover?	12
Chapter 4	Soul music	15
Chapter 5	A new dawn	19
Chapter 6	Interview	22
Chapter 7	A difficult start	25
Chapter 8	Adolescent anger	30
Chapter 9	Stuff those toys	34
Chapter 10	Surprising Bumble	37
Chapter 11	Early Christmas present	41
Chapter 12	The abbot's tail	45
Chapter 13	Stepping into the dark	48
Chapter 14	Who's fooling who?	52
Chapter 15	New surprises	55
Chapter 16	Special treat	59

Chapter 17	Really raining cats and dogs	63
Chapter 18	A dog's life	66
Chapter 19	Not just for Christmas	71
Chapter 20	Abbot, Tessa and Boutros	75
Chapter 21	Denise re-roled	79
Chapter 22	Outsiders	82
Chapter 23	Who's he trying to kid?	87
Chapter 24	Have car, won't travel	92
Chapter 25	Bumping into a blindy	95
Chapter 26	Socialising	99
Chapter 27	Streetwise	102
Chapter 28	Dog lore	105
Chapter 29	Before Abbot	110
Chapter 30	With Abbot	114
Chapter 31	Out on the town	118
Chapter 32	Show us your money	122
Chapter 33	You think I can't do it?	127
Chapter 34	He can see, you know	131
Chapter 35	Flashback	134
Chapter 36	Progress?	138

Chapter 37	The blind leading the sighted	142
Chapter 38	Soapbox	145
Chapter 39	Disabled, disadvantaged, abused	149
Chapter 40	Art lover	153
Chapter 41	Dark days	158
Chapter 42	Walk the dog	162
Chapter 43	Mixed messages	165
Chapter 44	We'll just write	168
Chapter 45	Onward!	171
Chapter 46	Bad reception	174
Chapter 47	Speaking for myself	178
Chapter 48	Facing my fear	182
Chapter 49	Why do I love him?	186
Chapter 50	The abbot's rule	188
Chapter 51	I owe you one	191
Chapter 52	My guardian angel	196
Postscript	Hope for the future?	201
Contact info	Quick reference contact list	208
Your story	Do you have a story to share?	210
The author	Who is David Lucas?	212

Foreword by Bernard O'Donoghue:

A glimpse into what matters

On the evening of Saturday, 24 May 2008 I was sitting in the Neville Hall at the Mining Institute in Newcastle-upon-Tyne, listening to the great singer-songwriter Allan Taylor. I remember it very particularly because I was in remarkable company in that audience: one third of the listeners were handsome, quiet labradors, golden or black, accompanying their masters and mistresses at this event in support of Guide Dogs for the Blind. Everywhere around us were images of light and sight. The institute's lecture theatre, we were told, was the first public room to be lit by electric light, during a lecture by Sir Joseph Swan on 20 October 1880. Stephenson's original miner's lamp is a treasured presence in that grand institution.

I was there to read poems. The obvious choice was Seamus Heaney's masterpiece 'At the Wellhead'. At the beginning of the poem the poet is listening to his wife:

Your songs, when you sing them
With your two eyes closed
As you always do, are like a local road
We've known every turn of in the past.

When his wife sings with closed eyes it reminds him of 'that blind-from-birth, sweet-voiced, withdrawn musician... our neighbour Rosie Keenan [who] knew us by our voices'. This poem returns to haunt me as I read David Lucas' wonderful, luminous, illuminating book about his experience as a sight impaired person whose life has been totally changed (it's tempting to use the word 'redeemed') by his guide dog Abbot.

By the way, I haven't used the words 'luminous' and 'illuminating' by accident. Both words have associations of light and sight, just as so much of our language does.

David Lucas tells us that image is everything. This is yet another reminder that words drawn from sight are everywhere. By a metaphorical bias in our language 'understanding' is made equivalent to 'seeing'. We say: 'I see what you mean' or 'I see your point of view'. But of course this is only metaphor. The great, medieval English poem *Piers Plowman* ponders the things of the world but then says 'Piers the Plowman perceiveth more deeper'. And that is how it is in *Stepping Into The Dark*. To see with worldly eyes is a great blessing, but it only involves seeing the surfaces of things. David Lucas teaches us that there are more important, deeper kinds of seeing. Fortunately for us, he is a magnificently gifted teacher who can be humorous, withering, emotional or factual.

It is hard to decide whether this wonderful book will be of greater help to people who are only just beginning to lose their sight or to the severely sight impaired – who we used to call 'blind' – or if it will be their loved ones who will gain most. I even suspect that ophthalmologists, opticians and GPs will gain an enormous amount from reading David's account, not to mention politicians and people who have no normal contact with the sight impaired. Certainly, this book will give hope to people who are experiencing sight loss by showing them how acceptance and constructive measures can change their lives. It will also help the sighted to understand the predicament of the sight impaired and encourage them to respond with greater sensitivity.

But it will do more than this for everyone who dares to explore these pages because this is a book about love and humanity. Of course, this is not so different from 'caninity', or 'dogginess', if you prefer. In these pages, Abbot the dog is often shown behaving with greater understanding and wisdom than most human beings. The memorable phrase that David Lucas uses to describe what this dog brought him is 'healing and peace'. We could all do with some of that. Above all, the book teaches us insistently that the way to cope with any trial in life is fight, not flight, tempting as the latter always seems to be.

There are all kinds of other insights in this wonderfully intelligent, thoughtful book, which is also such easy reading. Music is central because it is so crucial to the conduct and enjoyment of David's life. He raises the question of whether relative deficiency in one sense leads to higher development in another... The blind musician has been a reality as well as an icon in Irish history since the Middle Ages. The tradition begins with Homer who, as Yeats says in 'The Tower', 'was a blind man'. It is found in China and Japan and everyone knows of its presence in the Country and Blues traditions in the USA. Nobody could forget hearing (or seeing) the blind musician Ray Charles singing 'Take These Chains From My Heart'. Why, I ask – if it's true – is there such a connection between music and sight deprivation? And why is it so touching that it's a dog who ends up helping the author of this book with such grace and generosity and friendship? Why is there such power in this particular version of the relationship between person and dog, which seems to reverse the normal master-servant relationship?

When I was young I was very close to my farm dog Bran. Obsessively, I read stories about deep relationships between person and dog, *Greatheart: The Epic of a Shepherd Dog* (Armada Books 1964) being one of them, I seem to remember. But I never found a book which explored the link like this book does.

Here you will find a deeply moving exploration of the relationship of dependency and mutual reliance between a man and his guide dog. You'll find a great deal more than that, though. In this book we are very close to the absolute centre of the things of importance, to what life is about and why it is worth living.

Everyone should read this book. No one will read these pages without being changed by them.

Bernard O'Donoghue
Oxford University

Introduction:

My blockbuster?

My friends always told me I should write a book. I always found an excuse not to, but it was there, at the back of my mind. It was something I would get round to one fine day. Meanwhile, I imagined I would become the next Dan Brown and the book – *The Lowry Code* – would be my masterwork. I would become an internationally best-selling author. Fame and wealth were just round the corner.

Then life threw something unexpected at me – something I wasn't ready for – at a time when I least expected it. As a result, the political thriller I was going to write had to go on a back burner. But gradually I realised there was another story to tell. So this is the story of a stubborn man who can't see too well any more. Although there is absolutely nothing wrong with his hearing, he will often simply refuse to listen. He doesn't want to and you can't make him. That man is me, David Lucas, a man who has gradually lost more and more of his eyesight. I'm the hero of my book and instead of being tall, dark and mysterious, as I'd always intended, it turns out I'm rather short, fat and grumpy.

Life threw something unexpected at me...

This book will not always show me in a good light. Indeed, it will sometimes show me as a bad-tempered old fool, full of self pity and more than a little bitterness. You might ask why I would risk being seen in this way...

The world is strewn with obstacles.

Well, above all I wanted to give you an honest account of my experience of sight loss, warts and all. The world of the severely sight impaired (who used to be called 'blind') is strewn with obstacles, often placed there by sighted people who are simply unaware of the effect their actions can have on the life of a sight impaired person. You will hear me rant and rave and generally stamp my feet about these things and I know this may be difficult. At one point, I thought about removing all such material from the book and had gone as far as highlighting huge tracts of text, ready to delete them. Then I realised there would be very little left as I rather like ranting and in any case it would in no way represent my true feelings as they arose along this journey.

I eventually decided to give you the full version of my journey – including the tears and tantrums, the anger and joys – and let you form your own opinion. Sometimes what I say may surprise you. Sometimes it may make you sad. Sometimes it may shock you. I suspect it will even cause offence. (I don't really write off whole groups of people, as you might sometimes suspect... but I have made this mistake at various times in my journey.) Occasionally, my thoughts may give you a laugh. And I earnestly hope and pray that just once or twice they might inspire you.

By the way, in case you're wondering why this book isn't in large print, let me explain. This book is really intended for people who are worrying about their eyesight or who know someone who is sight impaired.

This book won't provide you with all the answers about sight difficulties because as yet I haven't found them. What I have done, however, is reach an accommodation with my sight loss so that I'm no longer at war with it. I'm now able to wear the label of a blind man and not feel embarrassed or hurt by it. It has taken well over 40 years to get to this point... Even if I had known years ago what I know now, I cannot honestly say that I would have done things any differently.

Through this book I want you to gain a sense of what life is like for sight impaired people in the UK in the early 21st century. People with sight impairments still face prejudice, abuse and ridicule on a daily basis, causing them to lead lives of segregation, isolation, fear and – all too often – loneliness. I long to see many things but more than anything I want to see a world where opportunity is open to sight impaired people on an equal basis. I'm sad to say, we still have a way to go.

If more sight impaired (and severely sight impaired) people are to achieve their full potential, then society needs to change. This will only come about when we're able to face the issues honestly, all of us together, sighted and sight impaired. This book is simply one man's attempt to create a debate about how that will be possible.

As a sight impaired person, life isn't perfect. But it can be such fun. And it really can be fulfilling and worthwhile. Sight impairment is bearable and it is possible to lead a full life despite it. Believe me, I do.

David P Lucas

David Lucas

Chapter 1:
Déjà vu

At first I think it must be a bad dream, a nightmare. I need to check. I tug at the hairs on the back of my hand. It bloody hurts. That doesn't happen in a dream. I must be awake then. Great. That's just great.

I'm trudging down a corridor in an old Victorian building, dragging my feet, trying to hang back, thinking to myself that these Victorians really knew how to build. They were the people that built all these buildings that were designed to intimidate little people and keep the plebs in their place.

Everything about this building makes me feel small and insignificant. The glazed tiled walls are closing in on me. The corridors echo memories of footsteps belonging to the lost and bewildered.

What am I doing in this horrible building? The atmosphere hangs in the air like the smell of damp leaves on an autumn day. The pain of all who have suffered here permeates the very fabric of the building. It oozes from the wood and stone and drifts through the halls, like mist on a November morning.

This is a cold place. A sad place. A place where too many dreams have been broken. Hopes dashed. It's like walking into a fog: before you know it, you're cut off. There's no way out. I'm filled with feelings of panic and dread.

I'm filled with panic and dread.

As I push open the huge oak door and step forward into that unknown territory, the world of the blind, I see my reflection in the brass doorplate. It's a look I know all too well: the look of a person who is desperate, frightened, angry.

As I enter, I see the waiting room is full. It's packed with people who, like me, have spent years in denial, afraid that their sight loss will be used as a weapon against them, so that they can be held back. These people are all wearing the same haunted expression of people who've spent too long on the run. They're desperate, like me. I know that look on their faces because I see it every morning as I peer into the shaving mirror.

After reporting to the receptionist, I sit down, comforting myself with the fact that I've managed to postpone this moment for years and years. I've had a good run but it's time to face the music. Sight loss is now such a big issue for me, I can no longer hide it from other people or – even more importantly – from myself. But the impulse to run away from the truth is still there, goading me.

This has been the pattern of my life so far, I must admit. In my younger days whenever anything happened to upset me, I used to lace up my trainers and take to my heels. I would run just as far and as fast as I could until I felt utterly exhausted. As I got older and I realised my eyesight was failing me, I would jump on a train and head off to another town, a couple of hours away, often without a by-your-leave from employers, family or friends. I'd then drink myself silly in the vain hope that drink would blot out the pain I was feeling. I'd be gone for days. Sometimes I wouldn't come back until someone came and found me. Even though I knew it was a horrible thing to do to people around me, including my wife Denise, I just couldn't face the alternative. Today feels like one of those days. I know I'm not going to be able to face this...

The seconds tick past. Needless to say, I haven't come willingly. I feel as if I've been dragged here, kicking and screaming, even though I'm actually alone. It's just that I have no options left... I've simply run out of ideas. Years of refusing to recognise what's happening with my sight loss have been driving a wedge between me and all those who love me. Their lack of understanding begins to wind me up and eventually sends me spinning into a rage.

You wouldn't believe the anger I've felt.

You wouldn't believe the anger I've felt and somehow I haven't been able to stop myself from lashing out at people. On a rational level I know it's not their fault (well, a lot of the time) but this is not a rational thing. It's a gut thing, which has been burning me up for years.

Now, even though I've decided I'm going to face the music I don't feel remotely happy about it. Boy, am I unhappy! I feel like I'm giving in. I'm damned if I'm going to do this thing graciously. Here I am, about to hand over control of my life to doctors, social workers and various other officials, who are going to lead me to places I don't want to go. These do-gooders are going to make decisions that aren't theirs to make. How are they going to affect my life? Will I still be able to earn a good living? Will I still be able to hold my own in the world? Will I be in control? I begin to curse myself for getting into this situation. I feel totally hopeless.

I watch the other poor lost souls...

I watch the other poor lost souls in the waiting room, who are just like me. We're all people who no longer have control over our own destiny. Poor sods. I hope you don't imagine I've been caught, though... On the contrary, I was the one to turn myself in. I was a master of disguise and something of an expert in the art of evasion techniques. They would never have caught me. Oh and don't go thinking I'm a criminal either! No, I'm just a man who has always believed that sight impairment is socially unacceptable, on a par with robbing old ladies. I've been made to see myself as a kind of public nuisance.

Suddenly, the receptionist speaks.

"You can go through now, Mr Lucas."

I obediently walk into the tiny little office and am instantly transported back to my childhood. It's like falling through a gap in reality. In my mind's eye I can picture my mother spitting on her handkerchief and rubbing the chocolate stains from my chin. (She would go on rubbing until the skin was red raw.) As I remember this I feel her hand on my back pushing me forward over the threshold and I can feel my feet slipping and sliding as I try in vain to resist.

I do a reality check in an attempt to pull myself together. My wife, Denise, used to be a sister at this hospital. For her it was simply a place of work, a building that held no terror. For me, though, it's always been a place of fear. Just stepping across the threshold instantly transports me back to the most painful parts of my childhood. Here I am, a 40-year-old man with the mindset of a six-year-old. Damn this place! And damn the circumstances that have brought me here.

Really, this building should feel like a second home. As well as my sight impairment, I was also born with a heart defect. So between the Eye Department and the Children's Cardiac Unit, I often spent long periods of my childhood in various parts of this hospital.

How is it that one building can rob me of all my adult faculties and return me instantly to my childhood? How come I suddenly feel I'm no longer in control? How come other people get to make all the decisions here? Why is it that my opinions are of no importance to anyone when I'm in this building? Why is it that every time I walk through that huge oak door I feel like a midget in a world of giants? It's like Lilliput in reverse. I'm dammed if they're going to tie me down.

A phrase from my childhood echoes in my mind: 'Shut up and do as you're told.' My neck begins to stiffen and I feel my shoulders hunch. Again I return to being a child with short trousers and little National Health glasses that leave deep grooves behind my ears. Here I am, a 15-stone six-year-old, about to face up to something I've spent more than 40 years trying to avoid.

A phrase from my childhood echoes in my mind: 'Shut up and do as you're told.'

Chapter 2:

Consultation

I'm still in childhood mode when I sit down in this woman's office. I look at her and know at once she's more than just a megalomaniac, she's also a witch. She reminds me of Morticia from *The Addams Family*, that satirical televised inversion of the ideal American family. I can picture this woman sitting in that big wicker chair from the TV programme. Of course, I know I'm being unreasonable but at this point in time, no one could change my mind.

The woman smiles sweetly. The six-year-old me clenches his teeth and waits for her to ruffle my hair. I promise myself that when her hand comes towards me, I'll bite her fingers. Nevertheless, I try really hard to force the six-year-old me back into the deep recesses of my mind. Making another big effort, I smile right back. Anything she can do, I can do better.

Morticia rolls her eyes at me. I roll them right back. I concentrate really hard and force my features into what I hope is my most withering look. I don't know why really because I've often used that look and to date no one has taken any notice of it. Why it should be any different today, I don't know. Time seems to stand still, the silence is numbing. It seems to last an eternity. I'm waiting for her to speak but when she finally does, I'm totally unprepared for what she has to say.

"I think it's time you thought about a guide dog."

My world explodes. The ceiling seems to be falling in. She's still speaking but nothing is getting through. All I can hear are the words 'guide dog' echoing in my head. Guide dog?

A fucking guide dog?! They're for blind people. What the hell is she trying to say? Is she crazy? Do I look like a blind man?

No bloody way is this going to happen. Do I look like a blind man?

A High Court judge inside my head booms out:

'DAVID LUCAS! You shall be taken from here to a place not of your choosing and be given a guide dog. Henceforth you shall be known as 'Blindy Lucas'. Children will laugh at you in the street. Middle-aged women in twin sets and pearls will coo over you. They will take you to the seaside and buy you candyfloss. You will be given a short-back-and-sides and a set of hand-me-down clothes.'

No bloody way is this going to happen. Every fibre of my being is screaming at me to run. Run, Dave! Just bloody run! But something is making me stay, although I have no idea what... Somewhere deep in my subconscious I know that this is right. Why, then in the days leading up to this meeting when I was imagining every possible scenario did I not hear the words 'I think it's time you thought about a guide dog'?

Someone's made a mistake, that's why. This bit is totally unscripted... and now is not a good time for ad-libbing. I feel so angry! I've never known anger like this. How dare she? This woman who's never met me before, who knows nothing about me or my life. She's trying to pin a label on me, a label that says 'BLINDY'.

Well, I know exactly where she can stick it and she's damn lucky I don't tell her. This will mark me out as disabled, the very term that started me running all those years ago.

I'm on the verge of telling her all this, when I realise how futile it is. Tonight, as usual, this woman will mount her broomstick and fly off over the rooftops of Newcastle, back to her home and family. She's just doing her job. This is simply routine to her. But that one simple statement has blown my whole world apart. How can anything ever be the same again? I think: Witch! You bloody witch.

I really need to get out of this office. I've successfully avoided this moment for over 40 years and now everything has turned to dust in a split second.

I stuff my hands in my pockets so that I can be sure not to punch anyone or anything and I stomp off down the corridor, right out of the hospital, half out of my mind. My philosophy has worked for me so far and it'll just have to work for me again: when things get too uncomfortable, just run! But running is a young man's game and I'm starting to feel my age. Even as I jog along in my clompy boots, I have to admit there is one very big fly in the ointment: I've promised my wife, Denise, that I'm going to face up to whatever's going on with my eyesight.

That one simple statement has blown my whole world apart. How can anything ever be the same again?

Chapter 3:

An image makeover?

Sight loss is the monster that's haunted the backwaters of my life for the 20 or so years that Denise has known me. The fear of blindness has caused me to live a life of pretence and terror.

> The fear of blindness has caused me to live a life or pretence and terror.

Because of my fear I've treated everyone with suspicion. I've always felt that my sight loss will become a source of mockery. For me, every new person I meet is yet another potential source of ridicule. No one has ever been allowed an opportunity to have fun at my expense. If there is Mickey-taking to be done, I've always been the first one there. I have to get my punch in first.

But every time I've done a runner like today (and believe me, there have been many days like this one) Denise has been left behind, wondering what's going on. I've heard of the 'fight-or-flight syndrome' and I feel like I've had a lot of experience of the 'flight' part. How has she managed to put up with my disappearing acts? Slowing my pace, I realise that now is the time to try out the 'fight' bit. But how can I do that? It certainly doesn't come naturally.

I really want this to work for Denise's sake, but I'm not sure I have what it takes to see it through. I have to try, though. I owe her so much! But can I pull it off?

Up until now it's always been so vital that no one should know the full extent of my sight impairment. A guide dog is going to put paid to all that. A guide dog will announce to the whole world: 'Hey! I'm vulnerable. Feel free to have a laugh.' Besides, I've never seen anyone running with a guide dog and I've never seen a greyhound working as a guide dog.

In our 21st century world, image is everything. This is the designer age, where image is king. All our possessions must carry the right label: we have BMW cars, Nokia phones, Nike trainers and Armani suits. We shop at the trendiest stores because everything we purchase and where we purchase it makes a statement about who we are and our standing in the world.

How can I step away from this world of image? Getting a guide dog would be far from cool. I feel I must resist it with every fibre of my being. After all, the problem is not so much *having* a sight impairment as being *perceived* as having one. I'll suddenly be disabled not just by a lack of sight, but by a negative stereotype that pervades the whole of society.

Till now I've thrown people off the scent.

And in any case how can I abandon all the years I've dedicated to the cause of hiding my sight impairment? Believe me, I've become very, very good at doing that. I've raised it to something of an art form, something I'm particularly proud of. It's always been imperative that no one should know the severity of my sight loss. I'm not alone in this. Ask any sight impaired person — we all do it. We memorise things that a sighted person wouldn't even turn a hair over: phone numbers, price lists, bus timetables, addresses... Many other trivial items are committed to memory so that we're not seen to be struggling in public.

Until now I've managed to maintain my elaborate scheme to throw people off the scent of the truth. Each morning I listen to the newspaper review on Radio 4's *Today* programme. I also buy a newspaper and scan the larger headlines and pictures. In this way I make myself familiar with the main stories of the day, even though it means using a magnifying glass, even though I keep losing my bearings on the page and even though I can't do it for too long. Then, when a conversation comes up, I feel able to contribute on an equal footing.

No one ever need know I can't read properly like other people. I'm pretty typical in this respect. We sight impaired people never knowingly place ourselves in a situation where we might be open to ridicule. We devise all kinds of fantastic excuses to make it impossible for other people to guess the severity of our sight loss. Personally, I've taken this to a whole new level.

Yet here I am about to make myself more vulnerable than I've ever been before in my whole life. I know I have to take this next step, but I feel far from happy about it. I was deadly serious about the promise I made to Denise because I knew our future depended on it. But that voice in my head is still urging me to continue running. Go on, Dave. GO ON! You can do it. Just get the hell out of here!

That voice is still urging me to keep running.

Chapter 4:

Soul music

A week passes. I stay at home. There are times when the urge to do a runner is strong but, thankfully, I manage to hang tight. Still, I do nothing as yet about the guide dog idea either for or against. Perhaps you're wondering why? I've asked myself the same question many times. I know I need to do something for Denise and all the other people who love me, but I feel paralysed. Am I feeling sorry for myself? Dead right I am! Do you have a problem with that? Sod everyone else. This is not about you, this is all about me. In truth, there are no laudable reasons that spring to mind for my non-action. My feelings are just a painful blur but a few song lyrics seep through to my consciousness as I lock myself away with my guitar...

Music has always been so much more than an interest to me. It's what keeps me sane in this crazy world. It often provides me with answers to questions which I don't even consciously know I'm asking. People often talk about music as the soundtrack to their lives. For me it's even more fundamental than that: music has been my life's road map. It influences all my decisions and guides me to new places – often places I'd never have dreamed of going to otherwise. For me, to be a spiritual being, it must be possible for a person to be affected by music. After all, music is the language of the soul. This is why it can often convey what would otherwise be unspeakable. For me, music can often express what's in my heart far better than words alone.

Actually, I even have a theory about this. I have no real evidence to back it up, but I still believe it whole-heartedly. My theory is that sight impaired people make special use of music and explore its deeper meanings even more than sighted people. Since we can't read facial expressions or body language so successfully, we pick up all our nonverbal clues via sound. Nuance is a language we're fluent in. Inflection and tone are our currency.

I often feel at a disadvantage not being able to pick up on cues that are purely visual.

In the sighted world, I often feel at a disadvantage not being able to pick up on cues that are purely visual. It's even easy to feel inferior or paranoid because it's like trying to conduct an argument when only your opponent has access to the full facts.

In the world of music, on the other hand, I feel I have the upper hand. This is my home ground, a place where I feel the odds are more stacked in my favour. This is largely why music remains my favourite art form. I prefer music to literature, art or movies. With music I'm on more than just a level playing field with the sighted world... I feel like I'm the one with the upper hand. Music has always been a safe haven for me, a kind of sanctuary and a place of retreat. Whenever I feel sad, lonely, upset, depressed or in any way troubled, the chances are I can be found listening to music or playing my guitar. When I feel like shutting the world out and telling mankind to go to hell, it will be music that brings me back out of myself. It provides me with the resolve to carry on.

It's nice to feel I'm sometimes gaining insights.

Denise has sometimes accused me of being a musical snob and to be totally fair to her, she has a point. But in the sighted world where I miss out on all the other nonverbal cues, it's nice to feel that sometimes I'm gaining insights that sighted people are missing out on. Sighted people have access to people's facial expression and body language. Meanwhile, I have all the nuance, inflection and tone of music. It's my true domain.

Over the passing years, many other interests and even passions have come and often faded away. Their remnants are stacked in boxes in the attic because I try to kid myself that one day I'll take them up again – even though we all know that's not going to happen. Music has always remained, though. There's no thrill greater than rushing home with a new CD and popping it straight into the player. I still love to hang about in guitar shops, dreaming of owning their many treasures. I surround myself with musicians too. Last night I mentally compiled a list of my mates and I discovered that only three of them were not musicians.

There has always been something about the setting of words to music for me. Words set to music become more significant, their meaning stronger. Words in song embed themselves in the mind, reverberate and echo. Loudon Wainwright III, one of my favourite songwriters and a well-known hellraiser and teller of the tallest of tales, once said he was incapable of telling a lie in a song. In fact, I often find Loudon's songs just too painfully honest. I find myself feeling embarrassed as if I've overheard something private. It's like reading someone's diary.

The music of songwriters such as Allan Taylor, Jackson Browne, Ray Davies, Dougie MacLean and many others has often been the only thing I've been able to cling to. Songwriters such as these have kept me sane at times when I was closer to the edge than I'd have cared to admit. I use their songs to relate to things that are generally unspeakable, not just focusing on the lyrics but also on the backing track, which can often speak to me far more deeply. The arrangement is very important to me... it's what conveys the artist's smile or frown. Because of the secret messages which I feel are communicated, I like to think of music as a secret language to which only a chosen few can have access.

I like to think of music as a secret language to which only a chosen few can have access.

It's not all positive, though. I often feel as if songs are ganging up on me. They point out my failings and shortcomings and, worst of all, they steer me in directions I'd rather not go. As I thought about this guide dog issue, I felt as if new songs were coming at me from all directions. Each one seemed to be nudging me, changing my course, pushing me forward. Most of my favourite musicians were coming up with song after song that seemed to speak directly to me. It was as if they knew I was facing a difficult decision and they were all determined to have their say. Bloody musicians. How did they know so much about my life? I was beginning to think they might all be spying on me.

Chapter 5:

A new dawn

One evening, I'm chopping onions to make chilli con carne. I don't notice that the white lead from the kettle is on the chopping board and I cut right through it. The next thing I know, there's a very loud bang and I come to sitting on the floor at the opposite end of the kitchen. I'm just beginning to realise what's happened when the doorbell rings. It's Dave Newton, an old friend, and he seems to take this electric shock business a bit more seriously than me. We have a bit of a row about whether or not I should tell Denise. In any case, I realise I need to summon up the courage to go back to my consultant and have her put me on the sight impairment register. Why did I run away from her when she suggested the natural next step? Perhaps I'm just not keen to step into the darkness...

I'm not at this point discussing things with a living soul – not my wife, my mates, or anyone else for that matter. No one shares my real thoughts and feelings. This is going to be all my own work, my grand gesture to Denise. It'll show her that I am finally taking my sight loss seriously. At last I'll be off the hook.

Of course, the main reason I'm not speaking to anyone about this is that I'm afraid they might hold me to anything I say. Before I make any public announcement, I need to be sure it's something I can adjust to and live with. At this point, I'm still not sure that's possible.

No one shares my thoughts and feelings.

I feel as if I was managing a few steps in the direction of acceptance when that witch went and mentioned a guide dog. That buggered everything up. I'd never considered this as an option before and I'm still frantically trying to buy myself some time. I'm not at all sure I'm ready to come out of the sight impaired closet in this most public of ways.

One evening I bring some work home and take a couple of new CDs into the study with me. Through listening to Allan Taylor's music, I'd come across the work of Dougie MacLean and I'd just bought my first Dougie CD, an album called *Riof*. I sit at my computer, pushing it into the CD player as I start to work. The words on my screen begin to melt. They're sliding down the screen, forming little puddles on my keyboard and I realise my cheeks are wet. I'm crying. Dougie has reached into my soul and one section of the song has broken me up completely. Instinctively, I know I have to notice this. I contemplate the words as Dougie sings...

Sometimes we search too deep. That's when the darkness feeds our fear. We turn away from one another in case we get too near. Me, I stand this mountain top... I shout so she can hear. And I know that she will find me. I know that she will find me, even if I vanish without a trace. Oh and though I'm running blindly, I know that she will find me, dancing with the shadows that I chase.

[From 'She Will Find Me'. Music and lyrics by Dougie MacLean. Published by Limetree Arts and Music (PRS & MCPS UK). Used here with kind permission.]

Running blindly? That's an understatement. I've been in total panic for years. All I've been able to do is flee. Sight loss is just too unthinkable. So I've been running, hiding and lying my way through many years until everyone who's close to me just can't stand it any more.

You just wouldn't believe how I do this. As well as swotting up on news stories and memorising key details, I also try and take in as much as possible of anything I do manage to see.

People are often surprised at the amount of detail I remember about a scene. The truth is that I store more detail in my memory because the next time I look at the same scene my sight may not be working as well as last time. I know I might never be able to see something again because my sight comes and goes. I look at everything as if it may be the last time I will ever see it.

I know if I don't stop running soon, I'll lose those I love. But running's become an automatic response and stopping won't be easy. I'm not sure I'm in control any more in any way. Yet no matter how far I've run, I always knew that deep down I wanted to be found. And until now, Denise has usually been the one to come looking. So why can't I just stand up and fight? Perhaps I'll give it a try... But it's going to be tough to give up and really hand myself in.

> If I don't stop running soon,
> I'll lose those I love...

Chapter 6:

Interview

Somehow I manage to make the right phone call. Then, a few days later I find myself in my front room answering questions from a lady from Guide Dogs – the Guide Dogs for the Blind Association (www.guidedogs.org.uk). It's now over ten days since my hospital visit but my temper has in no way cooled. The abiding memory I have of that day is of me forcing my clenched fists into my pockets in the vain hope that this will be enough to stop me hitting someone.

We begin to talk about long cane training and as we talk I begin to feel tears welling up in my eyes. I'm beginning to lose control and for that very reason I'm already beginning to resent this woman.

Doesn't she realise those long canes are the stuff of nightmares to me? As a child, I remember watching a blind man walking down our street using a long cane. I was standing at the bus stop beside a crowd of middle-aged women. Predictably, the man was dressed in hand-me-down clothes, with no thought for colour co-ordination. He had a really bad haircut and his face was spotted with little bits of toilet paper where he'd cut himself shaving. His gait was ungainly, his steps hesitant, and he seemed very unsure of his footing. I can remember the pseudo-sympathetic chorus from the women – 'Ah, isn't it such a shame?' – as the tap-tap-tap of his cane faded off into the distance.

This picture has stayed with me for years and something about it scares the living daylights out of me. Every time someone mentions blindness it's that picture that comes flooding back to haunt me. That picture is at the heart of all the running. It's this image that has fuelled all the lies and forced me into years of denial. There is simply no way I'm going to be like that man.

I'm not going to allow myself to be patronised. I don't need anyone to feel sorry for me. After all, I'm already doing enough of that for myself.

The very thought of that man with the white cane fills me with panic once more and squeezes the breath from my lungs. Nodding at the nicely-spoken woman, I imagine myself reaching down for my trainers, once more ready to run. This has become my instinctive response. After each escape I eventually find myself far away from home, wondering how I've got there. I realise I no longer have any control over this response... and here I am about to run again.

Suddenly, I see Denise's face, drawn with worry. She's seen me like this far too many times before and I know I can't do it to her again. I have to sit tight, so in my mind's eye I fumble my shoes back into place and try to force myself to sit up again. As I listen to myself speaking, I can hear my voice rising and I know I'm in danger of completely boiling over. I feel so damned angry! I want to throw this bloody woman out of the house. How dare she think of me as a blind man?! I don't look like a blind man! My haircut's pretty cool and my clothes are my own. To hell with her! I want to shout at someone but most of all I just want to break out of here and run.

I just want to break out of here and run.

My lack of participation must eventually get through to the woman because she suddenly suggests it's probably best if I'm left to calm down for a while. She leaves and I realise I've been really rude to her. Unwittingly, she's made me face fears I've been avoiding since my childhood. Boy, do I resent her for it!

She leaves and I realise I've been rude to her.

As I close the door on her I can feel Denise's eyes boring into my back. She's giving me the look – the look that says: 'You've gone too far!' I'm an old hand at embarrassing my wife and I've seen that look many times before. There's going to be humble pie on the menu for the next few days. Oh, bugger.

Chapter 7:

A difficult start

For a while after this I get lost in a red mist of rage. For as long as I can remember I've been strongly against the idea of a long cane. It's just not going to happen.

However, one morning soon after that interview Guide Dogs phone to invite me to their Middlesbrough centre for a three-day assessment. Long canes are not mentioned in the conversation. Despite this, I still can't bring myself to agree readily because the appointment I made with the social worker back at the hospital was really just a gesture for Denise. I wanted to show her how serious I was but it never occurred to me that things would develop in this way. On the other hand, pulling out now would mean a serious loss of face. I'll have to continue to go along with all these appointments and hope for a chance of escape somewhere down the line.

How have I got myself into this?

That's how I come to be sitting on the Middlesbrough bus a few days later. Imagine how I feel... Here I am about to spend three days with the twin-set-and-pearlies crew and they're going to give me a guide dog. It's been less than a fortnight since that bloody social worker suggested a dog and now I'm on my way to take a test drive. How in hell's name have I got myself into this? Lucas, you're a bloody idiot. My mind is racing. I feel bound by the promise I made to Denise but I still desperately need to escape.

All through the bus journey my mind is dragging up pictures from my childhood. I don't want to give you the impression that my childhood was desperately unhappy because it very definitely wasn't. However, my sight impairment was a constant source of ridicule and misunderstanding.

My eyesight was a constant source of ridicule.

Nowadays, what I experienced would be called abuse but it was just considered normal in the '60s. The ridicule I suffered at the hands of other children but also from some staff was left unchecked. My parents' deferential attitude to those in authority only made it worse. My mother was a teacher herself so she believed that the words of any so-called 'professional' – be they teacher, priest or doctor – must never under any circumstances be questioned, or worse still opposed. Consequently, members of all three of these professions were allowed to ridicule me because of my sight and I was forced to sit and take it like a good little boy. At best I was just told to grin and bear my sight difficulties. I carry the scars to this day.

Please don't misunderstand me here. I don't believe my parents were being unnecessarily cruel. They were simply products of their generation, just as I am a product of mine. Indeed, my own experiences as a Baby Boomer have given me a set of expectations that are not at all healthy, nor fair to others. As for my parents, they were brought up not to question their betters. They'd been taught to see difficulties in life as character forming. It was natural that they should expect the same from their son.

Although my parents' constant insistence that I was the same as other children was a great boost to my confidence and served me well in many other ways, the flip side was that it gave me a set of expectations which were unrealistic for someone with my condition. Unable to accomplish the same things as my brother and sister, I was left with the feeling that maybe I'd let my family down. And I was also left with the sneaking suspicion I was just a little bit thick. (Now you can keep your own thoughts to yourself. No one asked for your opinion.)

In any case, I did not share my parents' attitude about professionals – I've never been that deferential. I was born bolshy. I was never going to take bad treatment without a fight. I must have been around six or seven when I first started retaliating. Teachers saw my behaviour as disrespectful so I soon learned that standing up for myself would lead to trouble. Nevertheless, when I stood up for myself and fought back I at least felt that I was the one controlling things. For me that's always been, and remains to this day, a priority.

Because of my approach, I've spent a great deal of time at loggerheads with my family. This has been a great source of sadness and heartache for me. I have absolutely no doubt that my parents' reluctance to recognise my disability was well-meant, but it did mean I failed to get the help I was entitled to and indeed the help I needed. I suspect this was the norm in the '60s and there probably wasn't that much help available then anyway. I suppose the staff at the schools I attended simply weren't trained to deal with my impairment. I even doubt that things are that much better now, almost 40 years later.

Please don't think that the situation with my parents remains unresolved. In recent years we've reached a new understanding, which is a great source of joy to me. Actually, the writing of this book has helped greatly in that process. (An unexpected bonus that I had never foreseen.) My lasting regret is that for most of my life I was unable to communicate to them what a great sadness my sight impairment was in my life. I felt unable to tell them what was going on so they never knew the level of ridicule and abuse I was living with. I was embarrassed by it and therefore I refused to discuss it with anyone. Not talking about it has always been my strategy. I suppose I felt that ignoring it might make it all go away. Put your hands over your ears and whistle tunelessly... That had always been my best coping mechanism.

To give you an example of what I experienced, I remember walking across the playground at the age of seven. A ten-year-old boy jumped out in front of me.

"Hey, cross-eyed Clarence!" he yelled. "Don't look at me like that."

Clarence was the name of the cross-eyed lion in the TV programme *Daktari*, which was about a fictitious East African game reserve. Clarence was to become my nickname and would haunt me for years to come.

"Are you sorry for looking at me like that?"

I thought about that one for a couple of seconds and then I hit him, SMACK, right on the nose. Serves him right, I thought. Suddenly, there were people all around us and I was treading air. A teacher had grabbed me, lifting me clear off the ground. He frogmarched me straight to the headmistress's office.

This ten-year-old thug had started it but I was the one in trouble. Even at such a tender age there was something in me that would not let me just walk away.

The headmistress told me to hold out my hand. I got strapped. She demanded that I apologise to the boy. There was no way I was going to do that. He could go hang! When I refused, I got strapped again. Even so young, I knew the injustice of it and I made up my mind that one day someone would pay, just as soon as I was big enough.

I spent a long time waiting to be big enough. Once I was, a whole load of people did a whole lot of paying, most of whom had never done me any real harm in the first place. I was hurting, angry and miserable and I never like to be miserable alone.

I was hurting, angry and miserable and I never like to be miserable alone...

Chapter 8:

Adolescent anger

Trundling along on the bus towards the Guide Dog Centre I also remember my first few months at senior school. Every day was a constant onslaught of taunting and ridicule. In the end, I used to hide my glasses before entering the school gates and I spent my days frightened to look up at anyone in case they called me 'Clarence'. I refused to ask if I could sit at the front near the board, where I needed to be, as this would have drawn attention to me. (Why would I willingly invite further abuse?)

Eventually, because I was unable to see much of what was going on in class, my work began to suffer. Quite apart from the blackboard, I also had problems any time I was supposed to share a book with another classmate. (Unless I could actually control the book and hold it inches from my face, it was no good even trying to make out the text.) I even began to play truant from certain classes where the teachers thought making fun of me was great sport. The fear of being caught playing truant seemed much less of a worry than the fear of being ridiculed. I felt alone and victimised and the resentment began to build, a resentment that would follow me into adulthood and lead to all kinds of trouble later on.

I remember one time particularly when I was 12 years old and at grammar school. My teacher called me to the front of the class and asked me to read a passage aloud to the rest of the class. I raised the book until it was about four inches from my face and began to read.

"STOP, CLARENCE!" the teacher shouted. "If you read like that you'll go blind."

I tried to explain that in fact this was the only way I could read but before I got the chance to finish my explanation I was told to shut up and he insisted that I hold the book at arm's length. At this distance I could only make out about one word in three and I stumbled and stuttered my way through the passage.

By the time I was halfway through the whole class was laughing hysterically and then someone shouted 'Go on, Clarence!' That was the last straw. I threw the book to the floor and stormed out of the classroom. The teacher came storming after me down the corridor, roaring that no one ever walked out on one of his classes. Well, I thought, there's a first time for everything. When he eventually caught up with me he clipped me round the back of the head.

"One day you'll pay for that," I told him, so he hit me again for my trouble. Now there was definitely a score to settle. I stuffed my hands in my pockets to stop myself hitting him right back, a gesture of mine which has become a kind of trademark.

The day of reckoning did arrive, when I was 40. It was a long wait, but nonetheless rewarding. I was in a coffee shop in town when I bumped into my former teacher. He was wearing very thick, half-rimmed glasses and was struggling to read a newspaper. His head was buried deep inside the paper with his nose almost touching the page. Serves the old bastard right, I thought.

The day of reckoning did arrive when I was 40.

The temptation to pass comment was just too great. I marched up to him and grabbed his paper. I began tugging at it until his arms were fully extended.

"Do you remember me, you bastard?" I shouted.

Looking very confused, he replied: "No..."

"The name is David Lucas. Or maybe you remember me as 'Clarence'?" I could tell he remembered me now.

Suddenly all conversation had ended.

Suddenly all conversation in the rest of the coffee shop had ended and we were the centre of attention. That was fine. I was happy to have an audience. I'd waited for this moment for 28 years, so I was determined to enjoy it. It seemed only right that others got to join in the fun. Was it worth it? You bet. I did resist the temptation to clip him round the back of the head – but only just. With hindsight I wish I'd had the nerve.

This was the outcome of just one event in my childhood which made me resolve to reveal to no one the full extent of my sight impairment. After all, I knew only too well how much abuse and ridicule I would face if people really found out my situation. Nevertheless, covering up something as big as sight loss involved a huge amount of trickery and deceit and it was to bring me a whole new set of problems.

Even now, as I approach Middlesbrough for my three-day assessment, I realise that my plan is to sabotage the whole procedure I'm about to face. However, I also know that there is one big flaw in my plan: I've always been a dog lover and we have a golden retriever named Tessa.

Owning Tessa has taught me just how much love and joy owning a dog can bring.

Owning Tessa has taught me just how much love and joy owning a dog can bring. She's now an old lady of 12 and she's seen us through many difficult times. She was there when Denise's dad died. She just gently nudged Denise to let her know she was there. And she did the same for me through a period of ill health. Tessa has taught me that dogs can be sensitive creatures, attuned to our emotions and capable of great caring and compassion. I realise it's Tessa's fault I'm on this bloody bus... Bless her!

Chapter 9:

Stuff those toys

On arrival at the bus station I'm met by yet another of those nice ladies from Guide Dogs. She asks if I'd like to take her arm so she can guide me. This hasn't happened before and I'm certainly not ready for it. To say that I'm taken aback is something of an understatement. How could she possibly mistake me for a blind man?! I make another of those instant decisions that I'm so fond of: I'm not going to like this place. Once again, I force my fists into my trouser pockets and smile sweetly.

"Thanks, I'll be OK," I say. By now my jaw is beginning to ache from all my insincere smiles.

The lady turns out to be Lynne, who later becomes my guide dog trainer. Eventually, I develop the greatest possible respect, admiration and affection for her. But right now I just feel angry and have a sense that this woman embodies the enemy. My bottom lip is sticking out and my dummy has been thrown out of the pram...

Ten minutes later we arrive at the centre where the biggest shock of all is awaiting me. I am about to have my first real encounter with the BLINDIES and I am totally unprepared for the experience. Nevertheless, I'm immediately struck by the atmosphere of the centre. There's a tangible feeling of healing and peace, as if the very walls of the building are exuding the love of all the generations that have gone before. It makes the hairs stand up on the back of my neck. Damn this feeling! I promised myself I was going to hate this place. This should not be happening.

> Foolish as it might seem, it's never occurred to me there will be other sight impaired people here.

I'm taken to a huge common room, which is packed full of people with sight impairments. Foolish as it might seem, until this moment it's never occurred to me there will be other sight impaired people here. I've been so wrapped up in my own feelings. I don't perceive myself as part of this group and can't see how on earth I fit into this category. Someone's made a mistake.

I stand in the doorway with my hands in my pockets, unable to move, as if my feet are stuck to the floor. Crossing that threshold would be admitting my own sight impairment and that's simply not an option. I stay firmly put and say hello without entering the room. If I stay out of the room then I'm not part of the blind scene. I'm just a visitor here, passing through. Not a blind man. On a very physical level I'm not capable of stepping over the threshold. It's as if my boots are glued to the floor. As long as I stay outside the room I won't catch the dreaded Blindy Disease.

Suddenly, a memory flashes through my brain. Skinchies, I think. As a child, I loved playing hide and seek and 'skinchies' is a Geordie word children use when they're playing this game. No one can catch you while you have skinchies. Skinchies guarantee you immunity. They buy you time out. Boy, do I need time out right now! I'm not ready for any of this and I have no idea how to cope. The toys are well and truly out of the pram now.

Later that morning we begin our first session and we're introduced to Stuffy, a toy dog on wheels... a 'baby walker'. Immediately, I felt demeaned. I'm angry all over again and am far from cooperative. I used to have one of these toy pull-along dogs when I was three or four. Now, at the ripe old age of 41, they want me to start playing with one again. I don't bloody well think so!

It's quite difficult to put a harness on a toy dog with clenched fists, but I'm a talented guy and I manage it. By now, I'm chewing a hole on the inside of my cheek to stop myself saying something inappropriate. Nevertheless, I do find out a few interesting things about guide dogs. I learn that they're instructed to do quite complicated things with various short, learned commands such as 'Forward!', 'Butcher's' or 'Bus stop'. The command to cross a road turns out to be an interesting one because I learn that it's not the guide dog who decides when to cross the road, but its owner. (Of course, that's why there's an audio signal to cross, as well as the green man.) Having said that, it turns out the dog does have a lot of say in the matter too because if the owner gives the dog the command to cross when it's dangerous, it's trained to make absolutely no response. I also find out that the 4,600 guide dogs working in the UK have all learned to walk in a straight line in the centre of the pavement (providing there's no obstacle), stop at kerbs and wait for commands (to cross or turn left or right), deal with traffic and *not* turn corners unless instructed to do so. Reassuringly, I'm told they've also all learned how to judge height and width so that their owners don't bump their heads or shoulders. Hmmm.

Chapter 10:

Surprising Bumble

Eventually, later on that same day Lynne takes me out with my first-ever guide dog, a dog named Bumble. Bumble is a beautiful, two-year-old golden retriever bitch, very like my own dear Tessa. Someone is trying to win me over, knowing I have a soft spot for dogs that look like this. Well, it isn't going to work. I'm wise to this strategy and made of stronger stuff.

I desperately want to ruffle Bumble's fur and make a fuss of her but I know that once I do that the game will be up and I'll be getting a guide dog. That simply isn't about to happen. Lynne follows along behind us constantly nagging me to praise my dog but I resist again, so poor old Bumble gets none of the praise she deserves. Lynne carries on repeatedly nudging me in the back, telling me to praise my dog but I simply don't listen.

Little do I know as I stand on the kerb outside the centre that my life is about to change forever.

I'm convinced the whole thing is a waste of time and am on the verge of passing the dog back to Lynne and walking out on the whole thing. But then we come to our first junction and something special happens... For many years now I haven't been able to stand on the edge of a kerb without losing my balance and swaying like a drunk. This is a side effect of my condition and has led to a great deal of ridicule, leaving me feeling very self-conscious.

This has left me feeling very self-conscious.

Crossing roads has become something I fear not just because I can't see the oncoming traffic but also because I'm always expecting someone to make a wisecrack about the drunk about to fall off the kerb. I've even begun to plan routes so that I cross as few roads as possible, often taking routes that take me far out of my way simply to avoid crossing as many roads. This is a highly impractical solution but it's nonetheless become the norm for me. Journeys needed extra planning and extra time must be allowed.

But now, as we reach the kerb Bumble places herself at once between me and the edge of the kerb, forcing me back from the edge and freeing me from that swaying sensation. Suddenly, in one life-changing moment a guide dog has grabbed my attention. I'd never have thought such a thing possible. This was not part of the plan.

Later on, back at the centre, I sit down for my evening meal, ready to take a new look at things. This is my first meal with my fellow blindies and somehow it doesn't seem as bad as I'd always imagined it would. Around the table I see people who are vibrant, interesting, witty and intelligent. There is no sign of a dodgy haircut. They are just like me in fact: cool, trendy, lovable and modest. There is no sign of a hand-knitted, baggy jumper and no one offers to take me on a trip to the seaside. It's not at all what I've been expecting.

For years I've deluded myself into thinking I wasn't like these people. I've always refused point-blank to accept my sight impairment. It's never occurred to me as I've been about my business crashing into things and staring myopically at things for ages on end, unable to read them, that other people already perceive me as being sight impaired, irrespective of the impression I try to create. As far as I've been concerned, if you have no dog and carry no cane then no one knows. How wrong can you be? Yet for years that really is what I've truly believed.

Gradually, I start to realise that we each have very little control over how other people perceive us. What matters is who we know ourselves to be. Bugger! How could I have been so stupid?

Later that evening Lynne takes me out for a second session with Bumble. It's 6.30pm and since it's October it's already pitch dark, moonless and definitely a night when the old Dave Lucas would have found some lame excuse not to be out. I use various ploys to avoid facing the fact that on a night as dark as this I simply lose all confidence and become totally night blind... Perhaps it's too cold. Or I'm washing my hair. Or maybe there's this programme about dung beetles that I just can't miss.

But tonight here I am out in the dark with this dog, being followed about by this strange woman who keeps giving us instructions in a very loud voice. And yes, I've even been persuaded to wear fluorescent clothing. They told me it's for insurance reasons but I reckon it's just so they can get a cheap laugh at how uncool I look. I plod along, feeling cold, uncomfortable, embarrassed and frightened.

I'm about to take my third lesson. Bumble and I are settled at the kerb. Lynne says that when I'm ready I should give Bumble the command forward and cross the road. Until now, I've never been able to judge the speed of traffic and for years I've been crossing roads using my ears alone. The logic goes if you can't hear anything it must be safe. Of course, this is not a foolproof system and I've been run over twice because of it. I'm also used to being frequently screamed at by terrified motorists as I step off the kerb in front of them. (I must admit, this has almost been happening every day recently.) As Lynne explained to me earlier on, I've even been in constant danger of being run over by a milk float – let alone by a No. 57 bus.

I've been in constant danger of being run over by a milk float—let alone a No.57 bus!

I listen to the traffic and decide that the nearest car sounds far enough away to be of no danger so I give Bumble the command 'Forward'. Nothing happens. I actually feel her dig her paws in and refuse to move. Hey, I think, this dog is faulty. I want my money back! Then I hear Lynne behind me sniggering. I don't know what you're bloody laughing at, I think. I change the tone of my voice to what I think sounds a more authoritative one and once again I give Bumble the command to move forward. Still nothing. Not a flicker. This dog is definitely a dud. They can have her back. This whole guide dog thing is a waste of time. Then, very suddenly, I hear a roar as a bus thunders past, inches from my nose. Bumble had spotted it and had judged it too close for comfort. So no matter how many times the fool at the other end of the harness asked her, she was not going to move. Guide Dogs refer to this as intelligent disobedience.

Chapter 11:

Early Christmas present

Late that night I phone home to let Denise know how I'm doing and as we talk I begin to realise that my plan to avoid getting a guide dog is in complete disarray. My plan to sabotage my assessment has been sabotaged by Bumble herself. Bugger! In one day I've become totally taken with the idea. But now I have a new problem... I don't believe my sight loss is bad enough to merit a guide dog. I've met all these other people whose sight is far worse than mine and guide dogs are so expensive. Surely these people will come first in the queue and I myself will stand little or no chance of ever getting a dog? I hear it costs £39,000 to train up just one guide dog and each one only has a working life of seven years. To make matters worse, there's apparently no government funding – the whole thing relies on voluntary donations from the general public to Guide Dogs. Oh, bugger! This doesn't look like it's going to happen after all.

The next two days only help to reinforce just what a huge help a guide dog would be, but I still feel certain I won't get one. Apparently, it's not a question of how bad a person's sight is, it's a question of how much difference a dog will make to a person's level of mobility and independence and how well he or she can work with the dog.

On the morning of my last day I'm filled with dread because I know that Mark, the coordinator, is going to speak to me and he has the power to decide which people will get dogs.

To my amazement, Mark tells me I've been successful. I can't believe my good fortune. He tells me it'll probably take about a year to find the right match and as I'm still in a state of shock I reckon this will just give me enough time to get things into perspective.

I come out of the meeting wanting to do cartwheels down the corridor. They're actually going to give me a dog! It turns out I have to pay a nominal 50p for it, but Guide Dogs are apparently going to foot all bills for dog food and vet visits. I think we can probably manage the 50p.

Just ten days later I take a call from Sue at Guide Dogs. She asks if I'm sitting down and I know at once there's been a mix-up. Mark was wrong and I am not in fact going to get a dog. But it turns out I'm the one who's got it wrong. She asks if I'm busy the day after tomorrow as she's bringing this dog Abbot to meet me. If we both get on we'll start our training the day after and it'll take about five weeks.

I consider ringing Denise at work to tell her the fantastic news but I can't get my fingers to work. I can't speak and I can't raise myself from my chair. I'm in shock. What about the year I'm supposed to wait? I can't believe it. Only three weeks ago I was totally opposed to getting a guide dog. Now I'm about to become a true blindy. What's more, I like the idea... I *really* like it!

A key to my change in attitude, I realise, is that I've at last found people – the twin-set-and-pearly brigade, no less! – who understand my eye condition. I've discovered that nystagmus, my main eye condition, is not solely my own, but common to all nystagmus sufferers.

Until now no one had ever understood and I'd begun to convince myself that I'd just imagined the problems. Now, at last, my problems have been recognised as real. I've spent so many years searching for this understanding and healing and walking into the Middlesbrough Guide Dog Centre was a kind of epiphany for me. At last I was in a place where I didn't have to pretend. I could be myself. I didn't have to explain my sight problems to anyone and the building was kitted out especially for sight impaired people. After all this time I've found a haven... a retreat... a centre of healing.

I'm an emotional wreck and I laugh hysterically, but tears also pour down my face. In the space of three weeks everything has changed: from being violently opposed to any suggestion that I might have a problem, I've now performed a complete U-turn. What's most unbelievable is that I like all this change! So I'm a blindy and I actually like the fact. Eventually, I take a deep breath, pull myself together and make the call.

Denise cries and I cry some more. Then we laugh and finally we just panic. We're now in November, it's the run up to Christmas and there's lots to do: presents to buy, cards to write, parties to go to and families to visit. We finally decide that all of that can wait. This is a golden opportunity. It just has to be taken now and to hell with the consequences. In two days' time I'm going to meet Abbot and the day after that we're going to start training. I can't believe it's happening! Christmas is suddenly on hold. I feel sure Jesus wouldn't mind... After all, he's partly to blame because this is what Denise has been praying for. Santa's sending me a guide dog. Ha! He'll never get it down the chimney!

"He's a golden opportunity," I blurt out.

Before ringing off Denise asks: "Hey Dave, what kind of dog are you getting?"

"Oh... he's a golden opportunity," I blurt out, exhilarated. I don't know and quite frankly I don't care.

Chapter 12:

The abbot's tail

Two days later Sue arrives alone. Immediately I feel worried she's changed her mind. However, I soon hear that she's left Abbot in the car and only plans to get him out when we've got Tessa settled in another room. A few moments later Sue re-enters with this very excited, very young looking, black lab retriever.

"This is Abbot," she says.

My world changes instantly. He sits opposite me and grins. I'm immediately smitten. In fact, it's the beginning of a love affair. We've never worked together but I know at once that this is the start of something very special.

Abbot is fully aware that as a guide dog he is a cut above the rest. He has a way of throwing his head back that says: 'Go away. I have a job to do and I can't be bothered with the likes of you.' When I saw him walk into the room I could almost hear Sean Connery saying 'Hi! The name's Abbot. Double 'b', one 't'. I'll have one bowl of water, no ice.' His cheeky, full-of-fun personality shines through and I know he'll always be the boy for me.

We never thought we could love another dog as much as we do Tessa but Abbot has stolen our hearts already and this soon becomes a pattern with everyone he comes into contact with. If ever anyone asks us for the £39,000 it cost to train him, I'll have my house on the market in an instant. No one's ever going to take my boy away!

That night, our first night at the centre, I close my bedroom door and Abbot and I are alone together for the first time. Both of us seem nervous and apprehensive. I'm missing Denise and I'm sure Abbot is missing his puppy walkers. As I lie on my bed Abbot begins to cry a little. I call him over and he lies down on the floor beside me. He rolls onto his back and I tickle his tummy. Then I hold his paw and I honestly don't know who is comforting whom.

Only a few weeks ago I was so insistent that I wouldn't have a guide dog under any circumstances and now everything has changed. Now I feel I'm amongst friends who understand that some of us have been damaged by their past experiences. I find all these feelings quite unspeakable. In any case, I feel no need to explain myself. What's important is that I no longer feel under pressure to try and disguise my sight loss. I've spent years thinking that I'd find this feeling in a church or at some type of shrine, or even with some religious community. I finally find it at a Guide Dog Centre, the very place I've been running away from.

The next afternoon they bring Abbot back to my room and they tell me that from now on he's totally my responsibility. They teach me how to groom him and they give me instructions on how to keep him healthy with good feeding and sleep routines. It sinks in. He's mine at last.

A few days later I'm sitting at my computer with music playing in the background as usual. Loudon Wainwright III comes on with his song 'Homeless'. I think of my gran and know she would have approved of my decision to have a guide dog. She understood me in a way that no one else ever will. A few verses jump out at me...

He's singing about companionship and loneliness, about that sense we have of having a home somewhere in the world. He's singing about the façade we often present to the world when people ask how we are — how we lie and sometimes put on a brave face.

But now I can hear him singing about friendship and again I think of my gran. She truly was my very best friend and she gave me that sense of being at home—of *having* a home even. Nevertheless, like Loudon Wainwright in his song, I know I will somehow pull through. Somehow I'll get through the night.

I realise there's nothing to run away from.

Later on, as I lie in bed I gradually realise that in Abbot Gran has sent me a new best friend and protector. Now I realise there's nothing to run away from. Home is with Denise and Abbot and it feels like the safest place on earth, just like Gran's house always did.

Chapter 13:

Stepping into the dark

It's midnight on an early December night and I'm standing in the middle of a very dark field. There's no street lighting. There's no moon. To add to my delight, it's raining cats and guide dogs. Happy days!

The former Dave Lucas would never have come here. The very thought of it would have caused him to panic. But this isn't the old Dave Lucas. This is Dave-plus-Abbot and things are very different now. Abbot has safely guided me to this point.

Lynne, who's been standing discretely behind us all the while, suddenly drops one of her little bombshells. She wants me to let Abbot off the lead for a free run. Now I really am panicking. In situations of extreme darkness I am very disorientated. I would never have been able to negotiate my way to the middle of this field without Abbot. Now, this fool Lynne wants me to let him go. Is she mad? If he fails to return I'll be stranded here with no way back. Oh bugger. I really don't want to let him go.

Have you ever stood at the side of a racecourse and listened to the sound of a dozen highly tuned equine athletes thundering past? Well, that was the sound of Abbot as he thundered off into the darkness. In situations like this, ten seconds seem like an hour and a minute more like a week. I'm in total panic! As soon as he's gone I've got his whistle to my mouth, ready to recall him. Suddenly, Lynne grabs my wrist and shouts:

"Don't you dare!"

I don't. (You wouldn't either, believe me.)

She makes me wait for what seems like months but is probably only around three minutes. Eventually, she lets me call him in and I blow his whistle. Nothing happens. I knew it. He's run away. I've been right all along. Suddenly, though, quietly in the distance I can hear a low rumble. This grows to a thundering roar, just like those racehorses, and gets louder and louder as 40 kilograms of black lab hurtle towards me out of the darkness. Then the noise stops abruptly. Panic takes over once again but, unbeknown to me, Abbot has decided to take a leap at me from about three metres away. I hear a sudden whoosh of wind and then the full 40 kilos hit me smack on the forehead, nose first. I come to. I'm flat on my back in the mud with Abbot licking my face, his tail wagging like a demented helicopter.

I hear Lynne behind me, roaring with laughter.

"Well," she says, "at least he's come back."

I'm lying in the mud, laughing hysterically, with Abbot on top of me. She knew he'd come back. No one likes a smart arse, though, and as the laughter fades I can feel tears streaming down my face. I hope that Lynne can't see me. I've been such a bloody fool. I've spent years running away from this moment but now Abbot's here and I love it. I bloody love it. All those years wasted.

The next night Abbot and I go out on our own. We don't have Lynne and her great powers to fall back on. We're totally alone. We make our way to the edge of the field without any problem at all. As on the previous night, there's no moon and it's pitch dark. I'm even more scared than I was yesterday. Most frightening of all is the idea that there is no one with us if things get tricky.

I know I'm mad to be doing this and if I had any sense I'd go back to the centre straight away. But as you must have learned by now, sense is not my strong point. I stand there for ages, wanting to leave but needing to stay.

Somehow I have to know that what happened yesterday evening wasn't a fluke. I have to know it didn't just happen because of Lynne's great skill and expertise. I have to know that Abbot can be trusted, relied upon. If I'm going to place all my faith in this dog then I need to know that he's worthy of it and that he won't let me down.

Tonight it's just me and Abbot. I've never pushed myself this far before. This is the stuff of nightmares and this is my way of attempting to confront them.

I give Abbot the command 'Forward!' and we set off for the middle of the field. This is the easy bit. With Abbot by my side I feel totally confident. But what I'm planning to do next fills me with fear.

As we stand in the centre of the field, I slip Abbot's harness off but hold on tightly to his lead. Then I try to summon up the courage to let him go. In my pocket I finger the keys of my mobile phone and tell myself that if things go wrong I can always call for help. With a final burst of courage I unclip his lead.

In an instant he's gone. He doesn't even wait for a pat. Oh bugger. I'm totally alone. It's too dark to see my watch so I've no idea how long he's gone but it seems like a very long time indeed. (Remember? I can still see a bit. It's just not enough to be able to walk around confidently where I want, when I want, even in the dark. And my eyesight comes and goes.)

Eventually, I blow Abbot's whistle and wait. Then I wait... and wait a bit more after that. There is absolutely no sign of him. Then suddenly, like before, I can hear that low rumble as he begins to thunder through the darkness.

A few moments later I feel something heavy pressing down on my feet and I can hear a thump-thump-thump sound. It's Abbot's tail pounding on the turf like a jack hammer. I stand in the middle of that field sobbing uncontrollably. I give Abbot a big, big fuss, slip him a treat, replace his harness and we float back to the centre.

Being able to stand in the middle of any field in the dark, feeling completely safe, is a major life-changing experience for me.

Being able to stand in the middle of any field in the dark, feeling completely safe, is a major life-changing experience for me. For the first time I realise I'm going to be able to put my total faith in Abbot. For a long time I've been so afraid of being out in the dark alone that I simply didn't attempt it. Hey, that's going to change now! I feel Abbot's already beginning to give me my life back. Once again I'll be able to go to the pub or to a concert. Not only is Abbot going to guide me, he's going to reawaken my social life.

Chapter 14:

Who's fooling who?

I'm always amazed by the public's reaction to guide dogs and you wouldn't believe the things people say about these fantastic animals.

It's early in the morning soon after I first get Abbot and we're training. We're coming out of a shop and I hear someone say:

"Ah. Look at that dog. I think they're bloody marvellous, those guide dogs."

We turn to see two old dears walking behind us. Ken, the trainer who is with me this morning, gives me a nudge and says:

"Watch this."

At the kerb we ask Abbot to sit and Ken kneels down beside him. He then proceeds to give Abbot a great long list of directions.

"Abbot, I want you to go to the end of the street. Continue to the next junction. Then I want you to cross the road. I want you to turn left and keep walking to the end of the street. At the end of that street you'll come to a newsagent's. I want you to go in and buy a *Daily Mail.*"

At this point I give Abbot the command 'Forward' and off we go. In fact, Abbot has only registered that one word 'Forward' but I hear one old dear turn to the other and say:

"That's marvellous. Bloody marvellous."

This phrase has since become a catchphrase for me and Abbot.

One evening the whole class of 20 decide to go out for a drink. As we're mere trainees and not yet qualified, we're not allowed to take our dogs with us. It's generally decided that I should be the guide as I'm the one with the most remaining sight. On the way out of the gate I guide one young girl into the wing mirror of a BT van and I spend the rest of the evening watching the egg on the side of her head grow bigger and bigger. On the way back I even somehow manage to lose one member of our group. He is eventually found two hours later, wandering the streets of Middlesbrough in a very bad mood. For some unknown reason he blames me for this and hammers on my bedroom door when he gets back, demanding an explanation. Now I know that not only am I unsafe alone, I'm also not the person to lead anyone else into trouble... A good lesson to learn, but a terrible blow to my ego.

The next day during training, Abbot and I are standing side by side at the kerb waiting to cross when an approaching Transit van flashes its lights.

"Don't you dare move," Lynne bellows.

We stay put. Nevertheless, as I stand waiting I reflect that since it's a bright, clear day conditions couldn't be better for using the little sight I have. But I'm not man enough to take on Lynne so we stand still. Lynne's policy is to treat every day as if it's one of my worst ones and I gradually realise she's right to do this. By now the van has slowed to a stop and the driver is flashing his lights again. It's stalemate because there's no way I'm going to move with Lynne hovering over me. The driver becomes impatient and begins to toot his horn.

There's no way I'm going to move...

Suddenly, he gets out of the van and begins to walk towards me. As he gets closer I can tell he's a big guy, a builder by the look of him. He comes right up close and at first I think he's going to thump me. I'm just preparing to duck when to my great relief he puts his arms round me and gives me a hug.

He comes right up close and at first I think he's going to thump me...

"I'm really sorry, son," he says, thumping me on the back. "I feel so fucking stupid."

Maybe he's realised there's no point in flashing lights at most sight impaired people – they simply won't see. And could he possibly have guessed the flashing would have been a distraction to Abbot? Before I can say a word, he grabs my arm and marches me across the road without even asking if that's where I want to be. I can hear Lynne's laughter from the other side of the street.

Chapter 15:

New surprises

Soon after this, I'm training with Lynne again. She wants Abbot to get used to the idea of spending short periods on his own so I've left him in my room this afternoon and I've slipped off to the common room to have a coffee. I sit there nursing my drink, trying to resist the temptation to sneak past my room window to spy on him. After half an hour I return to my room to find Abbot standing with all four paws on the dressing table, admiring himself in the mirror. As his eye catches mine he has that 'Oh bugger' expression on his face as I say 'DOWN!' He skulks off to the corner where he lies for quite some time with that sad look that only a lab can give you – the one designed to melt even the hardest of hearts.

This takes me back to the time I stood in my bedroom with my guitar round my neck, wearing a tartan jacket and turn-ups. I was belting out 'Lola' at the top of my voice in what I thought was a great Ray Davies impression when suddenly in walks my mother. Even now, I can still feel the embarrassment of it, the redness creeping from beneath my collar and crawling its way up my face. I know exactly how Abbot felt when I walked in on him in the same way. Have you ever seen a black dog turn red?

Over the next couple of days, in trivial and profound ways, this black labrador continues to surprise me. Footbridges have always been a major problem for me. I'm not alone in this – the open staircases which lead up to them are a challenge for many sight impaired people.

One day, I happen to be travelling with Lynne across town and we're discussing this issue. As luck would have it we happen to be passing under such a footbridge at that very moment. Before I know what's happening, Lynne has pulled the car over. She lets Abbot out and gets his harness on and with a sense of dread I realise we're heading for the foot of the stairs. I can feel the panic beginning to rise but I know there's no point in arguing with Lynne, not when she's got that look on her face.

Many years ago I lost my balance on this kind of staircase en route to my friend George's house. I got such a fright I went into total panic and remained frozen to the handrail for quite some time until a passer-by spotted my distress and offered to lead me back to terra firma. For over 20 years since then I've been forced to make a significant detour whenever going to see George, so as to avoid it. I haven't been on a footbridge in all that time.

So here I am with Lynne and Abbot, standing at the bottom of the stairs. It's early December but I can feel the sweat running down my back. My mouth is dry and I feel like running.

"Just remember you're not the one doing this," Lynne says.

Thank God, I think. "No, Abbot is." My response sounds full of bravado but inside I'm thinking 'Oh bugger'.

Lynne's face is set. There's clearly no room for discussion, so off I set with Abbot. Within a split second I realise I'm not trying to judge the gap between those dreadful open stairs. Instead, I'm timing my footfall to the up-and-down movement of Abbot's harness.

Lynne was right. I'm not the one doing this, Abbot is. It's bloody marvellous! Just like those old dears said. For the next five minutes Abbot and I go back and forth over that bridge, five times.

Later when Abbot and I qualify at the end of our training, one of our first outings is a trip over the footbridge to George's house. I want to shout from the top of that bridge and tell the world how great it feels. I don't, though. Abbot and I know, and that's enough.

At the end of this footbridge is the cemetery where my gran is buried and as we cross the bridge, I swear I can hear Gran saying 'Good lad.' Actually, Gran's grave is a place of pilgrimage for me and in the months leading up to getting Abbot I've been looking for a sign from my gran that I'm doing the right thing.

When we get to the end of the bridge I take Abbot to Gran's grave so they can say hello. Abbot gives her headstone a lick and I have all the confirmation I could ever wish for.

Next morning we awake to find snow on the ground. Days like this have always been a problem as my balance is so poor. I'm prone to slipping and falling down so in the past I've broken bones, teeth and glasses. On days like this I usually just make my excuses and stay at home.

Over breakfast Lynne mentions that things might be difficult. Guide dogs use the straight lines of kerbs and verges etc. to find their way. When there is snow on the ground these markers are not always visible. I suggest we take the day off and begin again when the snow has cleared. However, as you might have guessed, Lynne's answer doesn't suggest any form of agreement...

I feel most impressed by how Abbot seems to sense my difficulty.

Once we're out in the snow I feel most impressed by how Abbot seems to sense my difficulty. Instead of his usual brisk pace he slows right down to compensate for my hesitancy. In areas that are particularly frozen he steps across me as if to warn me they're there. It's as if he's saying: 'Extra slippery bit coming up, Dad.'

Once more I think to myself, marvellous, bloody marvellous.

Chapter 16:

Special treat

The very next day my suspicions about Guide Dogs are confirmed. They really are one of those charities that like to take people on trips to the seaside. However, as Lynne comes towards me along the corridor I'm relieved to see she isn't wearing a twin set and pearls.

Okay, don't panic, I think. We're not going on a picnic and there aren't going to be any egg and tomato sandwiches. It's the middle of December so how can this be one of those clichéd seaside outings? We're simply going on a train trip to Saltburn, a small seaside town on the Cleveland coast. The idea is to see how well I cope on a train journey with Abbot.

Parking the car at the station, we head for the platform and make our way to the edge. The edges of platforms are even scarier to me than kerbs. After all, there's further to fall and the 10.15 to Manchester is likely to make a much bigger mess of me than the No. 57 bus. Kerb or station platform, I always get that same swaying sensation, so I'm expecting it again as I approach the platform edge. Abbot places himself in front of me again, though, pushing me away from the edge, away from danger. This really is bloody marvellous! Once we're on board the train I have my first experience of getting 40 kilos of dog under a British Rail seat. It's doable but by no means easy and Abbot is not happy about it. He has his huffy head on and is giving me withering looks from under the seat, accompanied by the occasional sigh for effect.

It's during this journey that I experience my first difficult guide dog situation with a member of the public. An old lady in the seat behind asks if she can give Abbot a sweet. Lynne explains to her that guide dogs are on strict diets since an overweight dog can suffer all kinds of health problems.

> **Lynne explains that guide dogs are on strict diets since an overweight dog can suffer all kinds of health problems.**

"Bloody stupid," the woman says. "He works bloody hard. He's entitled to a bit of fun. Miserable bastards."

I try to explain that there's nothing I would like more than to be able to spoil Abbot. She's right, he does work bloody hard and he deserves a fuss. But his health is much more important and I can't afford to allow him to eat rubbish.

As the train carries on towards the coast, Lynne and I carry on with our conversation. Then from underneath the seat I feel Abbot's lead begin to tighten and I soon hear the sound of munching. I realise the old lady has been sneaking sweets to Abbot under the seat. Lynne gives her the benefit of the arched eyebrow, but the lady doesn't seem too scared.

"We did explain why you shouldn't do that," Lynne ventures.

"Cruel bastards," the old woman shoots back. Clearly, she doesn't know who she's dealing with.

As we're getting off the train at Saltburn, I ask Lynne how I can be sure I'm getting off on the right side of the train. She replies that if the harness goes slack, then I'm obviously on the wrong side of the train. She proceeds to demonstrate by opening a door on the opposite side of the train and then she tells me to give Abbot the command 'Forward'. He refuses to budge and when I ask him a second time he turns and leads me away from the wrong door.

Once we're off the train we have some time to kill before our return journey so we set off in search of a coffee shop.

We're nicely settled at a table and Abbot is doing exactly what he's supposed to do, which is sit under the table, minding his own business. I drink my coffee and am busy munching on a sticky bun when once again I feel Abbot's lead begin to tighten. Lynne and I look under the table to find Abbot undulating, snake-like, across the floor, a butter wrapper stuck to the end of that cold black nose. Well, God loves a trier.

It's raining when we leave the coffee shop but there's still a little time to kill before our train's due. Lynne and I pull up our hoods and head for the beach, where we think we might let Abbot have a free run. As soon as he's free of his lead and harness, he's off. He winds himself up to full speed and heads straight for the sea. It's the middle of December, it's raining cats and guide dogs, it's freezing cold and Abbot still thinks it's a good idea to go for a swim. Well, that's my boy and I already love him. But just sometimes...

I already love him. But just sometimes...

Lynne and I stand at the water's edge watching Abbot head for Norway. That feeling of panic which has been held in check for the last few days is back again. Lynne tells me to blow his whistle and to my amazement he turns round and comes right back. Wonders never cease.

"I didn't expect him to do that," Lynne says.

"You didn't?" I pitch in. "I thought you were the bloody expert."

I haven't come prepared for Abbot's impromptu swim and I don't have a towel with me. I take off my jumper and use it to dry him off as best as I can. We get back on the train with one very wet dog and one very cold owner. Every now and again he gives himself a shake and everyone within 20 feet is given a soaking.

Abbot spends the entire return journey stretched out against a heater. Very soon the carriage begins to resemble a Chinese laundry as steam billows around our heads and the pungent smell of wet dog catches the back of everyone's throats. As Abbot lies there, steaming up the windows, he falls into a deep sleep and begins to snore loudly. People in the carriage begin to snigger and I feel like kicking him. I sit there jumperless and shivering, wondering what to do. Meanwhile, I can't decide if the rat-a-tat-tat sound I'm hearing is the sound of the train hurtling its way through the Cleveland countryside or the sound of my teeth chattering.

I look down at Abbot stretched out against that heater, steaming away, snoring his little head off, with a very smug look on his face. Bless him, I think. Oh well. Perhaps this time I can just put up with other people's reactions.

Chapter 17:

Really raining cats and dogs

Since it's the run-up to Christmas, down at the kennel block the staff are getting into a festive mood. They're wearing party hats and they're blowing up balloons. The kennel girls have also clubbed together and bought a Christmas tree – a really big one. It's standing in an old oil drum and it must reach about 12 feet off the ground. These are ideal proportions as the kennel block roof must be about 20 foot high. The tree is beautifully decorated with an abundance of toys and lights. It looks stunning when we first see it, but things are about to change...

As well as the many dogs boarded in the kennels, there are also a number of cats. The cats are employed as dog trainers: it's their job to familiarise the puppies with their feline counterparts. This is quite simply because working guide dogs must never allow themselves to be distracted by a cat. Cats used to form a queue outside the Job Centre for these vacancies. ('Room and board for the opportunity to take the puss out of dogs'.) Any cat would give his right paw for such a job.

Every time I go to the kennel block I'm struck by just how much the cats enjoy their work. With a taunting swagger and tails in the air they race round the rafters, some 18 feet above the dogs. This is the feline equivalent of giving the dogs the finger and the cats just love it. The dogs have been well trained and know how not to react. For the most part they manage very well and keep their base instincts in check but now and again the strain will get to one and he loses his temper. The sound of canned carols is then suddenly drowned out by a bit of barking, followed by some hissing, a bit of spitting and finally a yelp. Up in the rafters the cats chalk up another white line on their scoreboard.

Two days later I take Abbot back to the kennels to get him weighed again. As I walk through the door I feel my boot crunch on something. It's a bit of broken tree toy. I suddenly notice that the entire floor is covered with this debris.

When I get close to the tree I see there are only three or four toys left on it. Most of the needles have been shaken off, the fairy lights are bedraggled and the whole thing looks a total mess. As Abbot and I walk towards the scales something hits the back of my head. It shatters on the concrete floor and another tree toy bites the dust. The cats are stripping the toys from the tree and taking them up to the rafters to use as bombs to drop on the dogs. It seems there is no season of goodwill in the world of cats and dogs. After he's been weighed Abbot gives me a look which says 'I'll leave them alone for now. But one day, Dad...'

Denise, meanwhile, is feeling apprehensive. The last day of the training course is Family Day. She hasn't met Abbot yet and it's important that she does. Lynne and I drive to the bus station to pick her up. We leave Abbot in the car while we walk round to the bus stand. As the three of us walk back towards the car we see it's swaying backwards and forwards on its springs: it's Abbot, the canine helicopter, doing that thing with his tail. He's spotted his new mum coming down the street and boy is he pleased to see her!

Boy is he pleased to see her!

As Denise gets in the back of the car Abbot sticks that cold black nose through the dog guard and begins frantically licking the back of her neck. 'Hi, Mum!' he seems to be saying. It's the start of a great relationship. Their relationship really is very special indeed. He may be my working dog but he's his mum's little boy and when he's not working he's only got eyes for her.

Years later I find there's no point in setting off in the morning before Abbot has had his cuddle from his mum and there's nothing like the walk home again in the evening when he knows his mum is waiting for him. I'm often dragged at breakneck speed down the street so that Abbot can get home for his cuddle.

> I'm often dragged at breakneck speed so that Abbot can get home for his cuddle.

Chapter 18:

A dog's life

I graduated with Abbot on the 14 December 2001 and his certificate is proudly displayed on my dining room wall. I count it amongst my most valuable possessions and never miss an opportunity to show it off. You know those corporate training exercises where they ask you which one possession you would go back for if your house was on fire? Well, in my case, it's that certificate.

When I left the Guide Dog Centre I never dreamed for a moment I wouldn't see it again... But within six months it's been closed down. Apparently, it had to close down for lack of funds. I still miss it, as I know do many others. It played such a significant part in all our lives... It wasn't just a building. It was a place of healing and renewal, a place where many of us came to terms with our sight impairments and set out on a new adventure.

Since then, Abbot and I have become more and more of a partnership and his career goes from strength to strength. He is by now something of a celebrity. As I write, it's May 2008 and Abbot and I have been together for six and a half years. Abbot is about to celebrate his eighth birthday and I love him now more than ever. We've shared so much of our life together that I find it difficult to remember what it was like to go out without him. On the rare occasions that I do venture out alone, it's a very strange sensation to have nothing to do with my left arm, the arm I work Abbot's harness with. I keep looking under tables to see if he's OK and reaching down to ruffle a head that isn't there.

Abbot and I are now so much part of the scene that many people know me simply as Abbot's dad. Do I mind? Far from it, I consider it an honour. Nevertheless, Denise does get a little concerned when people stop us in the street to say hello to Abbot, knowing perfectly well who he is. As we walk away she'll ask me who it was and I have to admit that I have no idea. I don't count – I'm only Abbot's dad. Sue from Guide Dogs warned me that this type of thing would happen and she was concerned that I might draw unwanted attention to myself. I already had Tessa, though, and she was a very popular dog on the local scene, so I wasn't particularly concerned. Actually, even Tessa couldn't have prepared me for the magnitude of Abbot's fame but it's no price to pay for the joy of being out on my own in complete safety with my best mate, Abbot, by my side. All the panic I felt when I was on my own has completely subsided now and I feel totally confident, thanks to this wonderful dog.

I now know why celebrities are surrounded by so many flunkies and hangers on. There's a certain kudos to be had from simply hanging around with a superstar. I know because I'm Abbot's No.1 flunky.

Having Abbot has made me think far more deeply about relationships... I come from a Roman Catholic background and I even started training for the priesthood in my youth. Throughout my education I was taught that animals don't go to heaven and until Abbot's arrival this was a subject which had never exercised my mind. Now, though, I realise that things are different. Years have passed and I've given the subject a great deal of thought indeed.

Most people who meet Abbot make some comment about Abbot and Costello but for me there is a much more obvious comparison. For a long time I've been interested in Celtic Christianity and the idea of being led by an abbot has always had a huge significance for me. Following someone, or spending time with them, is often a way of acquiring new knowledge or skills. I know this because this is how I learned how to play the guitar. (Because of my sight impairment I was never able to read from sheet music and play at the same time.) I began to hang out with other musicians some 35 years ago... can't quite remember how it all started. I realised that if people spend enough time with experts most of them find that some of the skill rubs off on them. They pick up answers to questions simply by hanging around with these people.

This is how it's been with Abbot. The more time I spend with him, the more I feel I'm learning. Spending time with Abbot has taught me much more than I ever learned in the Catholic seminary. He's teaching me about the nature of faith. And it makes me think there must be a place for him in heaven too.

In case you're not with me on this one, let me explain a little... Scripture says there is no greater love than to lay down one's life for one's friends (John 15:13, New Living Translation). You may argue that this doesn't apply to Abbot because he's a dog. But do you want to be the person who tells him that?

On two occasions Abbot has put himself in danger in order to protect me. 'Yes,' I hear you cry, 'but was Abbot aware of the danger and did he choose it willingly?' My answer is a very emphatic 'yes'. Abbot has an innate sense of danger and usually spots it long before I do.

On the first occasion I was late for a meeting and panic had taken hold. Abbot and I got to the kerb and Abbot sat down and started waiting patiently, unlike his foolish owner. I listened and couldn't hear anything so I gave the command 'Forward!' Nothing happened. I asked him a second time and once again he refused to move. Sod this, I thought. If I don't get across this road and to the station for my train I'll be late. This meeting's important! Ignoring Abbot, I stepped off the kerb. Before I knew what was happening, Abbot stepped in front of me and marched me very briskly back onto the pavement as a car swerved round us, horn blaring. Abbot gave me his hurt look, the look that says: 'You know, you really should have more faith in me, Dad.' To my shame I knew he was right.

The second time Abbot and I were standing on a traffic island in the middle of a very busy road. Don't worry, I wasn't going to be stupid enough to step off the kerb again. In the distance I was aware of some boy revving his hot hatch racing car. Suddenly, Abbot turned me through 180 degrees and marched me back to the side of the road we'd come from. As I stepped back onto the pavement I heard a terrific crash as the boy racer mounted the kerb of the island and crashed into the bollard. We'd been standing there only a second ago. I knelt down and hugged Abbot. He simply shrugged and set off down the pavement to find a safer place to cross.

So in case you're wondering, when you have a guide dog, how do you know it's safe to step off the kerb? The answer is, you don't. You have to place your faith in your dog and trust that he'll make the right decision and not allow you to cross when it's unsafe.

Faith means hurling yourself into the unknown, putting all your trust in someone who loves you...

I know of a sighted vicar who was taken for a blindfold walk with a guide dog and he point-blank refused to cross the road in blindfold. For me this is a very telling tale and says exactly what Abbot has taught me about faith. Faith means hurling yourself into the unknown, putting all your trust in someone who loves you. Abbot has not let me down yet. If there is a heaven where Abbot won't be allowed in, then frankly I don't want to go in either.

Chapter 19:

Not just for Christmas

Christmas 2001 was the best Christmas since my childhood. I hadn't been this excited since coming downstairs to find a shiny new train set.

Abbot was the best Christmas present that anyone could have wished for and what did Abbot get for Christmas? Well, on Boxing Day we were walking down a street in our neighbourhood when he came across a turkey carcass that someone had dumped in the gutter. 'Happy Christmas', Abbot must have thought. He picked it up in his jaws, then continued to work by the book all the way home. I couldn't get him to let go of the turkey and Denise had to prise it off him when we got back.

Christmas came and went and represented a break in our training schedule. Then along came the New Year with a new set of challenges for the three of us. Abbot had to be exposed to a whole load of new experiences... experiences such as the Tyne & Wear Metro, the Shields Ferry and the articulated bus to the MetroCentre, the enormous shopping and leisure centre in Gateshead. He also had to be introduced to all my regular haunts: the library, the doctor's, the butcher's, the supermarket, my local pub and, above all, the local music venues.

There were many weeks of learning new routes. This was a tedious task but one that paid great dividends. Most of our regular routes are now so embedded in Abbot's mind that I only have to give him a key word and he'll take me to my destination.

If, for example, I leave my front door and give Abbot the key word 'Library' he will take me straight to my local library.

Now, six years on, I realise just how intelligent Abbot is. Let me give you two recent examples of how Abbot is constantly thinking things through, weighing up situations and making informed decisions.

On the way to our local newsagent's there's a place where the pavement floods whenever it rains. From the wall of the building across the whole of the path, right to the kerb, a huge puddle forms. To a guide dog a large puddle is an obstacle, an obstacle he must guide his owner round. As far as Abbot is concerned the puddle might be a hole, which his owner could fall down. This particular puddle, covering the entire width of the pavement, meant that Abbot would have to step off the kerb into the gutter to avoid the obstacle. Guide dogs are trained to step into the gutter to avoid things such as when there are workmen in the street. However, it is drummed into all guide dogs that this is a last resort. When they do go off the pavement into the gutter, they fit in tightly to the kerb and as soon as they are past the obstacle they step immediately back onto the pavement.

So one rainy day, I leave home and give Abbot that magic key word 'News' which means 'Take me to the newsagent's'. Halfway up the street Abbot makes an unexpected right turn. Now we've been together a long time and we've learned to trust each other entirely... So although I don't understand why Abbot is making this right turn I decide that I'm just going to go along with it and trust that he knows something that perhaps I don't.

So we carry on and I begin to understand what Abbot is doing. He's taking me to the newsagent's by going round the block in the opposite direction, thus coming to the newsagent's from the opposite direction and avoiding the puddle altogether. Abbot had worked it all out! He must have thought 'It's raining, that huge puddle will be there, so we'll go the other way.'

Very recently, the same thing happens again. I get off a train in Leeds during an episode where the little sight I normally have suddenly leaves me and I can feel the panic beginning to rise. Here I am in the middle of a strange, unfamiliar town, unable to see at all. I can't find my way out of the station, let alone to my destination. I try to attract the attention of some of my fellow travellers but they carry on rushing past. In sheer desperation and totally unsure if it will work, I turn to Abbot and give him the command to find a taxi. We set off and make many twists and turns. Once or twice Abbot seems to pause while he finds his bearings, but eventually we come to a stop and Abbot sits down. I am aware of someone standing next to me so I ask him if he knows where the taxi rank is. He tells me we're already in the queue and what's more Abbot has brought me straight to the head of it!

Abbot has taken me straight there!

Even on a normal day, Abbot exercises enormous judgment and skill on a moment-by-moment basis. Although he's very well qualified, believe it or not he's never studied geometry. So when he looks at a gap he's probably not thinking 'Now I'm about 25cm across and Dad's about 90cm, so let's see, that makes 115cm. We'll have about 5cm to spare.' Guide dog trainers guess that in the mind of a guide dog the owner and dog are one. So as far as Abbot's concerned, he's a very unusual creature who has six legs, two arms and only one good pair of eyes. What's more, these six legs, two arms and one good pair of eyes work together effortlessly as one unit. Existing as this unusual creature, Abbot has a good idea of how wide he is.

Existing as this unusual creature, Abbot has a good idea of how wide he is.

All this makes me realise we're a true partnership. I'm able to place all my faith in Abbot and he won't let me down. He is constantly thinking about how to help me. I can't begin to imagine life without him.

Chapter 20:

Abbot, Tessa and Boutros

Actually, the biggest worry Denise and I had when Abbot first arrived was that he and Tessa wouldn't get on. Tessa was the golden labrador we'd taken in as a rescue puppy some years before. She lived on for most of Abbot's first four years with us and mostly we needn't have worried. Nevertheless, theirs was a quirky relationship and not without its moments of tension.

Long before Abbot's arrival, Tessa had established a set of favourite places, all round the house, where she could get some sleep. Sleeping was what Tessa did best. Whenever I remember her face, it always has that 'just-woken-up' expression on it – half grumpy, half confused.

Whenever we had to leave Tessa at home alone for a short time she would head straight for the landing to catch a nap. When Abbot and I returned she'd appear at the top of the stairs, hair all over the place and staring short-sightedly at us. The look on her face clearly said 'Do you mind?! I'm trying to sleep up here.'

Her favourite spot for a snooze was always the rug in the hall. Tessa came to regard this rug as exclusively her property. When we purchased a new hall rug the biggest consideration was whether Tessa would like it. Both the old and new rugs were always covered in her hair and no matter how many times we ran the Dyson over them, the hair would reappear within what seemed like seconds. Every morning when I came downstairs I would retrieve the rug from under the radiator, which is where Tessa preferred it, and put it back in the centre of the hall. Moments later, Tessa would follow me down from her nightly watch on the landing... As she passed through the hall she'd shove the rug back to her preferred location, under the radiator.

Abbot sometimes used to get involved in these little territorial disputes. Whenever he was feeling annoyed with Tessa he'd take himself into the hall and plonk himself firmly in the middle of her rug. As she stomped past him, I swear I could hear him laughing.

Abbot also used to assert himself in other ways. For example, sometimes he'd make a hell of a noise with a pink, squeaky ball, which used to get on everyone's nerves. Still to this day (long after our poor Tessa passed away) he will sit in front of the bookcase where his toys are kept and stare at them. He'll then look from Denise to me and swivel his head back to where the toys are. He's got a huge collection of toys but this pink ball has always remained his favourite, mostly I suspect because it annoys us all so much. It used to bug the 'you-know-what' out of Tessa. Abbot would sit as close to her as possible and then squeak it as loudly and as fast as he could. This was torture for Tessa and she'd look at us as if to say 'Have you never heard of sleep deprivation?' Eventually, even Abbot wouldn't be able to stand the noise any longer and he'd wander out of the room in search of some other mischief. Once he'd gone Tessa would grab that ball and set determinedly about removing its squeak. Unbeknown to Abbot, Tessa was very good at this so by the time Tessa left us Abbot was up to his fifth ball, without him ever knowing. One day, I used to think, the shop will stop stocking them and then we really will have a problem.

I can relate to this because when I was a child I used to boast to my school friends that I had the same goldfish that I had won at a fairground some eight years before. I was in my 20s before I found out that I had, in fact, had four goldfish during that time. Each time the fish died my parents had searched local pet shops looking for a fish that looked the same as the previous one. They obviously cared about me so much, I really don't know why I didn't talk through with them my worries about my eyesight. When they read a first draft of earlier chapters of this book they simply said: 'But why ever didn't you tell us? If only we'd known.'

They obviously cared about me so much...

Getting back to dogs, Abbot and Tessa would both await Denise's homecoming each evening with great anticipation. One night this caused a slight incident. Abbot was trying to tick Tessa off and had taken up position on her rug in the hall. In retaliation Tessa had taken up Abbot's usual spot at the top of the stairs. Abbot was facing up the stairs sticking his tongue out at Tessa and she was facing down the stairs scowling at him. This had been going on for several hours and the offer of Bonios and several much loved toys could not coax either party away from the impasse. I was just contemplating inviting Boutros Boutros-Ghali – the Egyptian expert in international relations and peace studies – to come in and mediate and I was wondering if I had enough milk to make tea for all those blokes in blue berets when the front door opened and in walked Denise.

Hostilities were at once forgotten.
Tessa almost threw herself down the stairs.

Hostilities were at once forgotten. Tessa almost threw herself down the stairs to be the first to greet her mum. At which point Abbot decided to stand up and say hello to his mum too. The two dogs collided and Tessa was sent skidding across the laminate floor.

This was only the beginning of the trouble. For two weeks afterwards they spent all their time staring at each other from opposite ends of the room.

I was just on the verge of getting old Boutros and the boys round when something curious happened... I went next door to see my neighbours and when I came back I found them snuggled up together on the rug. Dogs, eh!

Chapter 21:

Denise re-roled

So far this has all been about dogs and me but I have to say that owning a guide dog hasn't only affected my life... It's affected the lives of everyone around me.

Before Abbot came along, Denise had spent the previous 20 years of our relationship as my unpaid sighted guide. Overnight she became redundant. She had guided me up and down stairs, kept me safe when crossing the road and guided me through busy shopping areas so that I didn't bump into anyone. More than that, she'd spent a lot of time worrying when I was out on my own. Was I safe? Had I got lost? Had I bumped into anyone? Had I had a fall? All of these questions and many more would play on her mind while I was out alone. She would call my mobile to make sure I'd reached my destination. She'd call if I was running late to see if I was OK.

When Abbot first arrived she began calling because what she thought should be a short journey seemed to be taking a long time. I had to explain that now I need to allow extra time for all the people who want to stop me to make a fuss of Abbot.

Now that I had Abbot and a huge amount of new-found confidence, I didn't always appreciate that Denise could not just 'switch off' her sense of worry. When she phoned me now I would get short-tempered and complain that of course I was OK – I had Abbot, didn't I?! But while I'd been given weeks of training and had learned to put my trust in Abbot, Denise had been given no such induction and didn't yet know for herself just how safe I was. Worrying was what she'd done for 20 years and I was asking her to suddenly switch off and put her trust in a mere dog – a dog that she loved but a dog whose capabilities she didn't know first-hand.

As far as Denise was concerned, she was still my principal carer. She was the one who looked out for me and kept me safe. It was her responsibility. So having Abbot was a difficult adjustment for both of us. It didn't happen overnight and caused more than one or two arguments as we both struggled to come to terms with our new roles in this situation and our new sense of identity. Somehow I wish my guide dog training could have involved her, so that we could have made an easier transition. After all, it wasn't just me who was going to be affected, it was going to be a big change for her too.

We were out at a function one evening and I over-heard Denise telling someone that 'we' had a guide dog. My first thought was that he's not 'our' guide dog, but *mine*. However, as I thought it through I began to realise that Denise was perfectly right in saying that he's 'ours'. After all, he's changed both our lives and is loved and cared for equally by both of us. A few minutes later I found myself standing next to a friend of Denise's. She told me she'd just been talking to Denise and mentioned that Denise had said 'I've got my husband back now.' I was so overcome by this that I had to go and stand in the car park for a while until I'd fought back the tears and regained my composure. She was perfectly right. The old Dave had been missing for quite some time. Abbot had found me and given me a new life. Bless him.

He'd found me and given me a new life.

Abbot brought just as many changes to Denise's life as he did to mine. For example, when Denise's mum became seriously ill, suddenly – and quite unexpectedly – Denise had a new source of support. Abbot stuck to her like glue. He would sleep on the floor on her side of the bed and every so often would give her hand a lick as if to say 'Don't worry, Mum.' It was clear that since we'd adopted Abbot as our responsibility, he'd decided to reciprocate and take complete responsibility for us too.

So on the whole the good outweighs the bad many times over, but there are still aspects of owning a guide dog that couples need to be aware of. None of these things had ever occurred to us as we set out on this wonderful adventure. I remember the days Denise and I could hold hands as we walked down the street. Now I encounter so many obstacles on my way down the street that I often need both hands to work Abbot. There are many pavements that can't accommodate the three of us walking side by side. It's now a rare thing for Denise and I to walk hand in hand and we both miss that a great deal.

Also, we often feel our intimacy intruded upon by the fact of having Abbot with us. The public have such an interest in guide dogs that many of them feel they have a share in Abbot. Imagine that you're having a light-hearted argument in the middle of M&S. You know the kind of thing... 'No, you can't have beef burgers, chips, beer, crisps and chocolate instead of salad for lunch.' The row is just reaching an enjoyable climax when some stranger sticks his face in yours and asks if he can stroke your dog. You must be sure you're ready for this kind of thing. Denise and I weren't but we're fast learners and we soon got the hang of it.

Chapter 22:

Outsiders

More than anything, owning a guide dog has changed the way other people relate to us. I found this very embarrassing at first. The centre where I'd done my training was not in my home town. That meant I'd been anonymous there, so there was much less scope for embarrassment. At home, I had to get used to having Abbot under the spotlight of people who knew me: neighbours, friends and family. I have never felt so self-conscious as I did at this time. And other people's reactions were interesting...

Some people had previously not known about my sight problem nor had they needed to know and often I still didn't want them to. Nevertheless, it's quite hard to hide when you have 40 kilos of black lab guide dog beside you. I felt very uncomfortable.

People we've known for years, who are well aware of my sight problem, suddenly started behaving differently. Sometimes it was funny, sometimes annoying and sometimes it was just downright hurtful. I have one friend that I used to go out for a pint with who found the attention that Abbot attracted very embarrassing. He no longer enjoys going out to the pub with me as much as he did before. We've retained a certain level of friendship but things are by no means the same.

One of our neighbours had an altogether different reaction: he refused to believe that Abbot was a real guide dog. On one occasion he told another neighbour the dog mess outside her gate came from Abbot. (Impossible, I can assure you. This is something a guide dog will never do. They only spend on command, and never in the street.) Another day he stood in front of me in the middle of the road holding up his hand, demanding that I tell him how many fingers he was holding up. I showed him two and walked away. My sight may not be all it should be but I still know what an idiot looks like. To this day he takes great delight in telling anyone who'll listen that there's nothing wrong with my eyesight.

People who knew about my sight loss but who had previously made no allowance for it suddenly started opening doors for me, helping me across the road and being generally over-attentive. In reality the only thing that had changed was that I had a guide dog. My poor sight had never worried them before.

There are others out there who will address my dog and never exchange a word with me. They tell their children to look at 'the lovely doggy' without ever thinking that this might make me feel uncomfortable. They tell them he's here 'to help the poor man see'. They never think to lower their voices and it doesn't seem to occur to them that their words might be causing me any distress. Sometimes, instead of making comments they just stare or start patting Abbot, without even asking. Then there's my personal favourite: the shop assistant or receptionist who will ignore me and ask the person with me what I want. I'm a big lad and very hard to miss, yet sometimes it would seem as though I was invisible.

Then there are the people who don't even notice us. I remember one time when Abbot and I encountered two gentlemen blocking the pavement. They were deep in conversation and totally unaware of our presence. I asked

Abbot to stand and said 'Excuse me' to the gentlemen. There was no response and they didn't move. I tried again in the same polite way, but still got no response whatsoever. After a third, equally unsuccessful attempt Abbot put his head down, pushed his shoulders out and ploughed his way through them. When we were past them Abbot stopped and looked back. He fixed the two men with a very stern glare which started at their toes and worked its way up to their heads. Then suddenly Abbot threw his head up and gave his tail a flick as if to say 'You're not worth bothering with' and set off on his way again. As we'd been waiting for the men to move I'd been concocting some very rude things to say, but Abbot's look had said all of those things and a whole lot more besides.

"Well done, son," I said. "I couldn't have said it better myself."

Finally, there are the people who are quite openly rude. For example, once when Abbot and I were walking down the stairs to our local Metro station I said to Abbot 'Tickets, son', which is the command I use to get Abbot to take me to the ticket machine. A lady behind me immediately piped up:

"Look at that! The dog even buys his ticket."

Another time, as Abbot and I were approaching the local library, a complete stranger suddenly accosted me...

"Excuse me," the lady said. "You do know that's a library, don't you?"

"Yes," I replied, aiming for a patient tone.

"Then why are you, a blind man, going in there?"

"Because the dog's books are overdue," I replied.

"You know that's a library, don't you?"

That reminds me of my favourite guide dog joke. A man takes his guide dog to the cinema to see the latest Harry Potter film. All through, the dog leans forward, apparently glued to the screen. As the lights go up a woman sitting behind the man leans over and says:

"Excuse me, but during the film I couldn't help noticing how interested your dog was. Don't you find that odd?"

"Well, yes," the man says. "He didn't like the book."

I also have to mention that there is the occasional time when people go out of their way to stand up for me. I had only had Abbot a few weeks when we bumped into Maxi, who is a comedian and old friend, outside a gig. I couldn't resist the temptation: I made Abbot sit and as Maxi passed by I put out my hand and said:

"Penny for a blind man, sir."

"Fuck off. You'll only drink it," Maxi said.

An old lady across the street heard this and didn't realise that Maxi and I were old mates... so she started belting Maxi with her umbrella and berating him for the way he'd spoken to me.

Another time, Abbot managed to completely astonish some friends. A group of us had gone along to a concert at the Newcastle Opera House – to see Maxi and his comedian partner Mitch. I was the only sight impaired person in our party but I was also the only person who happened to know the way. We'd arranged to meet under the clock in Newcastle's central railway station and planned to make our way to the theatre from there.

Abbot and I set off in the lead and I noticed that at every junction Abbot would stop and check that the rest of the party were still with us. Needless to say, this has endeared him greatly to the other members of our group.

Abbot and I set off and I noticed that at every junction Abbot would stop and check that the rest of the party were still with us.

Chapter 23:

Who's he trying to kid?

By now you may be wondering how I manage to see and be blind all at the same time. I won't give you a complete medical explanation – I wouldn't understand it and you'd be bored rigid. I will give you a brief outline of the facts, though, and a description of how my sight loss impacts on my life.

I was born with the condition called nystagmus, which I've mentioned before, which is characterised by an involuntary movement of the eye. In recent years I have also developed both macular degeneration and retinitis pigmentosa. All three conditions have seriously reduced my vision, which is getting worse each year. The effects on my life increase as my sight degenerates. The specialists have given me no long term prognosis because it's unusual for someone to have these three conditions together. This means that as well as living with the effects of my conditions, Denise and I also have to live with not knowing how bad things will get in the future, all the while having no idea of the timeframe it might all involve.

At the moment, the depth of my visual field is greatly reduced in my right eye and I can only distinguish dark and light in my left. One of the strange side effects of my combination of conditions is that often things I know to be square and true such as a door or window frame can appear to be leaning heavily to one side. More than once I've often put my hand out to lean on a door frame that wasn't where I thought it was and have consequently ended up sprawled on the floor.

Often I can be walking towards a door which appears to be leaning heavily to one side, and then as I'm almost on top of it, it appears to move in the opposite direction. This sudden perceived change can cause me to lose my balance. In other words, my vision is now giving me faulty signals that I can't trust as accurate, so it's all very disorientating.

My co-ordination is poor for the same reason. If I'm trying to pick a cup up, I can see the cup handle but because of the way my sight distorts the image the handle is very often not where I perceive it to be. This explains why I usually miss the cup completely when I put my hand out to pick it up. My poor depth perception means that I can't judge the height of things like stairs and kerbs. This also badly affects my balance and I now find that without Abbot I can't walk in a straight line. Rooms full of tables and chairs such as pubs and restaurants are a big challenge because I find it very difficult to judge gaps when furniture is close together. And this is all *before* having a beer, not afterwards!

My vision can vary from day to day and even throughout the same day. I can leave home with my sight performing quite well in my good eye. This can change mid-journey and problems may arise. My vision may also be affected by emotional and physical factors such as stress, tiredness, nervousness, or unfamiliar surroundings. Now I have Abbot this is not such a frightening experience because I am no longer solely dependent on my own resources.

My vision can vary from day to day.

On top of all this, I have what is known as a 'null point'. This means that by looking to one side or the other of an object I can achieve a point where my wobbly eye movement (the nystagmus) is reduced and vision improved. This is why sitting to one side of a computer screen or whiteboard may help. Adopting an unusual head posture also helps me to get the best from my sight. In other words, I might often seem downright odd when I'm looking at something. As a child and teenager this was a great source of ridicule and I'm still sensitive to comments about it to this day.

I may seem to be staring at someone when in fact I'm looking at something else entirely. As a young man I got into many a fight after people wrongly accused me of staring at them. Nowadays my problems are more personal: I get backache because I have to sit in an odd position, pressing my nose into my computer screen, and my computer monitor always has a sticky mark where my nose has been pressed. But at least I can still manage to use my PC.

I am light sensitive and good lighting of the right type is very important. There is some evidence to suggest that LCD lighting can cause people with nystagmus serious problems, such as temporary blindness, drowsiness or even blackouts. As a result, if a car approaches me with LCD headlights on (which are becoming more common) I simply can't focus for several minutes after it's passed.

I'm no longer able to read small print and I have to use large print which is at least 16 point. Even at this size, reading is slow and can cause me to suffer dizziness and a loss of balance. Often when I get up from my desk after a long period of reading, I find myself stumbling into things.

Of course, most of us have never really analysed how we read. I have a theory that we don't actually read each individual letter or even every word. Words such as 'and' and 'the' have a shape which is familiar, as do the vast majority of other words. I believe we recognise them instantly by their shape so in a way we don't actually *read* them. The only words we really read are the less familiar ones whose overall shape is new to us. I believe it's because of this that many people with a recent sight impairment still manage to read quite well.

I imagine the same applies to recognising people. I find it much easier to recognise someone very well-known to me from a distance because of their overall shape and the way they move. For example, I can stand at our garden gate and recognise Denise coming towards me from a reasonable distance. I can't see her features but since I know her shape, gait and even the sound of her footfall I can be reasonably confident when I call out to her that I'm right. Nevertheless, even with someone as familiar as Denise, I've come unstuck and called out to someone who wasn't her at all.

This ability to recognise well-known people has its pros and cons. One neighbour noticed me waving to Denise from a distance and was offended that I didn't wave to him from the same distance. Apparently, he'd tried waving at me from the same distance on several occasions, but I'd ignored him. He'd assumed I was being standoffish. I tried to explain that although I'd sometimes been aware of someone waving, I had no idea who it was or if they were waving at me. I had long since learned that waving at total strangers in the street can lead to all kinds of problems. Try it for yourself, if you don't believe me. Mind you, when someone gets abusive or punches your lights out, remember it was all your idea and you never heard about it from me.

In recent years, I've talked about these issues with many sight impaired people and I've discovered I'm not alone in experiencing these things... How many people do you know, I wonder, who are experiencing similar things, without you ever realising?

According to the RNIB (Royal National Institute for Blind People – www.rnib.org.uk) 100 people start to lose their sight every day in the UK. (This figure is based on the number of people who eventually register as sight impaired per year. People within the RNIB also generally believe that for every person on the register there are a further two who simply go unregistered.) Around 50% of problems would be preventable through the use of the correct glasses, contact lenses or cataract surgery (but few people have regular eye tests). Overall, about two million people in the UK are thought to have significant sight loss, most of them 65 years old or older. Younger people are also affected, though, and it's thought that around 25,000 children have problems with their eyesight in the UK. Despite these large numbers, in March 2006 only 364,615 people were registered as either severely sight impaired (i.e. blind) or sight impaired (i.e. partially sighted). Not surprisingly, perhaps, 70% of people with sight problems have other disabilities or long term health problems too. What *may* be a surprise is the fact that sight loss is increasingly due to obesity and diabetes. For this simple reason the RNIB predicts that sight problems will dramatically increase over the next 25 years.

Chapter 24:

Have car, won't travel

A typical teenager usually goes through many rites of passage. For me, the biggest ones were being picked for a football or cricket team, passing my driving test and getting my first car. Of course, because of my sight impairment I never got picked for any sports teams. I did somehow manage to get through my driving test and got a car... but of course, I wasn't able to drive for long. This meant the initial rite of passage was a bit of a non-event because it could never lead to the series of special cars I dreamed about. Much of my heartache and pain can be explained by these gaps in my life and I suppose they were at the heart of all the running, deceit and anger. And the negative feelings remain unresolved to this day. They haunt my dreams. They taunt, tease and goad me into losing control. They're the monsters which keep me awake at night.

During my childhood, no one would talk about these things with me and I grew up thinking I would have the same opportunities as my peers. I thought that all the things they could achieve would be just as open to me. But then, as I actually went through my teens it began to dawn on me that this was not the case. Nevertheless, it was hurtful that no one ever bothered to ask me how I felt about it and I certainly didn't feel I could raise the subject. I was hurting badly but I bottled up my feelings... and this unexpressed pain would make me defensive and abusive later on in my life. Looking back, I realise that everyone concerned was just too frightened to raise the subject.

An awkward silence began to grow, leaving a huge hole that everyone danced around but no one would talk about. I suppose they thought it might go away, but it never did. It just festered and festered and I grew more and more bitter.

My dad and my brother are both car buffs. I followed in their footsteps, dreaming of sports cars and Land Rovers and not imagining for a moment that it would never happen. No one had the courage to tell me it was unlikely I would be able to drive for long and until I was 17 it had never occurred to me there would be a problem. Loving cars as I did, I always assumed that one day I would pursue my dream. After my first car I'd go on to get better and better models as I progressed through life. But I now know that few people with nystagmus ever pass a driving test and even the few that do, like me, can't always continue for long.

Nothing in my life thus far had hurt me as much. I was a car nut, I loved being out on the road in a fast car with some loud music belting out of the stereo. To me there had never been anything quite so exciting but I knew my days were numbered.

I was bitter, hurt and looking for trouble. Nothing else about my sight impairment has affected me so deeply. I often encounter people who own cars that I would covet and yet they're not true car buffs and to them their cars are just another possession. This makes me so angry. I know people with wonderful cars and yet they never seem to go anywhere. I want to scream at them. Some of us long for the opportunity to just get in a nice car and drive.

Some of us long to just get in a nice car...

I don't think I ever got over this...

I don't think I ever got over this and I'm not over it yet. I feel so bitter about this one issue and although other scars have healed this is still an open wound. Perhaps this is because the car was always a symbol of freedom and independence for me and I've always felt that it was unfairly taken away well before I was finished with it. Even writing about the experience now, I can feel myself getting angry and upset. My head tells me that I'm over it but my heart yearns for a fast car and the open road. I still love wandering around car showrooms and watching *Top Gear* and *Formula 1* on TV. I'm now trying to live the dream by proxy.

As for the football and cricket, I often feel this is why I ended up becoming a musician. Since I was never going to excel at sport I took up the guitar. While all my friends were wrapped up in sport I was gaining a head start on the musical front. By the time they discovered music, I was years ahead of them so I was always in demand as a guitarist. I was the best guitarist in my school by virtue of the fact that I started years before anyone else. They were all too busy playing football. It was great to finally do well at something. But as far sport was concerned, it's as my friend Allan Taylor wrote:

Some dreams are carried away on the wind and never dreamed at all.

Chapter 25:

Bumping into a blindy

As I've said, I do still have some sight on most days and actually most sight impaired people do (contrary to popular belief). You might find this out to your peril if you bump into one.

I was on a train one day with Abbot when two teenagers sitting opposite were making two-fingered gestures at us. I lent over and suggested that maybe they should stop. They both looked very shocked and when they asked how I knew, I told them Abbot had told me. Needless to say, making fun of someone who appears to be blind, when in fact, they have a little sight, is not going to win you any friends.

Making fun of someone who appears to be blind is not going to win you any friends.

A minority of people with sight impairment can only distinguish light and dark and others a bit more than that. Some have no central vision, while others (like me) have no peripheral vision. Some see a patchwork of blanks and defined spaces. Others see everything as a vague blur. (I've got friends like that. Actually, it has nothing to do with sight impairment but a whole lot to do with the delights of the local brew.)

Some people are officially called 'sight impaired' and some are designated 'severely sight impaired', which, in some cases, can mean totally blind.

Fewer than 10% see nothing at all.

Surprisingly perhaps, fewer than 10% of those registered as severely sight impaired see nothing at all. This usually comes as a surprise to sighted people. When they see either a cane or a dog they tend to assume the person can see nothing whatsoever. But as the first few chapters of this book may have shown, people who cannot get around without these aids may still have some vision left.

There are so many eye conditions that can lead to serious problems that I can't list them all here. Some people are born blind or with reduced vision, some suffer sight loss through accidents and others simply lose their eyesight as part of the ageing process. The effects vary widely depending on the condition, its progress and how the person is coping at that point in time.

If you come across someone who seems to be having problems seeing, the important thing is not to find out what they've got or how bad it is, but to focus on behaving appropriately, so you can avoid causing offence or further problems – and so that you can actually provide some help.

Let's imagine you see a man who appears to be having difficulty seeing and you want to be helpful. First of all, talk to the bloke. Trying to anticipate his problems without talking first can cause hurt and offence. So don't lead him across the road without first asking a) if he needs your help and b) if he actually wants to cross the road in the first place. And after asking if he needs your help, also ask him what *kind* of help he needs, so you can help him as an individual.

If he wants you to help him cross the road, he'll probably want to take your left arm. Reassure him you'll keep half a step ahead of him and that you'll tell him about any kerbs or steps, etc. And if he asks you for directions, give useful instructions involving precise words. (For example: 'Go down this street and turn left at the next junction.') Specific directions are a lot more helpful than vague descriptions like 'over there'. And remember that pointing is of no earthly use to a blind person at all.

While you're with this bloke, don't treat him as if he's got some kind of infectious disease. He's just an ordinary person who happens to be sight impaired. He doesn't need your pity – beer, chocolate or money, maybe (only joking) – but pity, almost certainly not. Definitely don't go on at him about the 'wonderful compensations' of sight impairment. His sense of smell, touch and hearing and for that matter his sense of humour probably did not automatically improve as his sight deteriorated. There may have been some changes, but you can't assume there were. He's just an ordinary bloke.

If you're looking for something to talk about, consider avoiding the subject of blindness altogether. After all, it's an old story to him and he probably has just as many other interests as you – so why not try and find something you have in common? In other words, just talk normally, using an ordinary tone of voice. (Why shout? He's probably not stupid. And why ask his friend about him? Why not speak to him directly? Whatever you do, don't try to talk to him through his dog.) Just talk to him normally.

Consider avoiding the subject of blindness...

Don't be afraid to use everyday expressions which refer to sight such as 'Look' or 'I see what you mean' and don't worry if you ask him if he saw a program on TV. This kind of talk is part of our language and he probably won't want you to put him into some kind of politically correct crèche. And for goodness' sake don't ever call a visually impaired person a 'VIP'. This is horribly patronising and will almost certainly cause offence. My usual response to the term 'VIP' is 'FU2'.

In the end we're only talking about sight impairment here – it's not as though I come from Sunderland. (OK, OK! I know it's a wonderful town, with a fantastic football team.) Just don't treat me as if I've got some terrible disease because what I've got isn't catching. And as I've said, for your own safety, remember that I might still have enough useful sight to deliver a blow accurately.

For your own safety, remember that I might still have enough useful sight to deliver a blow accurately.

Chapter 26:

Socialising

Let's imagine you really do get friendly and you decide to have a drink with this person who can't see as well as you. If you're in a pub or a restaurant then clear directions to available seats will probably be much appreciated. (If you're ever lucky enough to be out with me, remember it's your round and mine's a Guinness.) If you're going to eat together, offer to read the menu out loud but don't try and choose a meal for your new friend and don't cut up his meat. He's blind, not underage. Most importantly, don't take the piss out of him.

Now, you may not be surprised to hear that one person who read an early draft of this book was very offended that I included language people had used to insult me and my reactions... It so happened that this reader is a friend and she came along to dinner with me and Denise and a group of friends over Christmas this year. Four big lads sitting at the table next to us spent the whole evening pretending to be blind. When I got up to go to the loo, they groped their way along behind me, laughing as they went. Our friend was amazed.

"Now you know why I get so upset," I told her.

If you should ever invite a sight impaired man to your home – a real one, not one of those fakes – it's probably a good idea to show him the bathroom, cupboards, windows and light switches too. This will help him become orientated, just as you do yourself when you look around. When you move from room to room, always leave doors either completely open or completely closed.

A half-open door is a hazard because it's confusing to someone who can't see very well. (You wouldn't believe the number of cuts and bruises I get from walking into half-open doors. This problem of mine has everything to do with my sight impairment and nothing to with my Guinness intake.) Last, but not least, if you leave your friend alone while you go off to do something, make sure you leave him near something he can touch, such as a wall or table. He'll probably feel very uncomfortable and disorientated if you leave him in an open space.

Beyond these basics, always be considerate. For example, if you happen to notice a spot or a stain on your guest's clothing, tell him about it privately, in the same way as you would wish to be told yourself. In other words, in this and other matters, treat any sight impaired person with the same respect you would wish to receive if you were in the same situation yourself.

Now for a warning... You may need to be especially sensitive, patient and understanding. Good-humoured jokes about the person's eyesight or difficulties getting around might not be taken well. I'm often told by sighted people that they've already tried to engage with a sight impaired person but they've had what can only be described as a negative response. I would urge you to remember that many sight impaired people suffer abuse from the public on a daily basis and it is the grind, grind, grind of this that can sometimes put a sight impaired person on the offensive. Also, remember that many sight impaired people haven't had great educational opportunities so they may not possess either good communication skills or confidence.

In case you're not sure what I mean when I say you need to be sensitive, consider what provoked me, one fine evening down the pub, when I was in my late 20s. Two guys at the bar were giving a young lad a hard time about his glasses, saying they looked like jam jar bottoms. I felt my hackles rise instantly, even though my friends were telling me this was not my fight. They'd almost convinced me to walk away when I heard one of the blokes call the man 'Clarence'. That was it. Something snapped inside me and reason flew out the window. I was back at school and these guys were taking the piss out of me. Before I knew what I was doing, I had one of them lying flat on his back on the bar room floor, with me standing on his chest, demanding an apology. I had to be dragged away by my friends before it got any more ugly. As I said, you may need to be especially sensitive, patient and tolerant.

You may need to be especially sensitive.

In a way it makes sense if you have a hard time when you spend time with a blindy. After all, facing up to sight impairment is a very difficult thing to do. Although it may seem obvious to you that it's best just to get on with things, the loss of eyesight may not be something that any one individual has come to terms with. This may mean they're particularly touchy.... I know because I've been there myself. If you catch me on a bad day – which, thank God, is much less likely nowadays – you may not get a great response from me either. But even if I'm grumpy, I'll privately appreciate any efforts you make, I promise.

Chapter 27:

Streetwise

You wouldn't believe some of the things people do that cause untold problems for sight impaired people. I'm sorry if you know about these already but there are still too many people out there who haven't got the message. Please feel free to pass it on...

Imagine the problems litter presents. Just picture me being helped out of a minibus by a nice sighted person. She tells me she'll see me back at the same spot in an hour. Not only do I have to believe that Abbot will be able to help me negotiate my way round all the lampposts, bollards, people, buildings and bus stops – to mention just a few of the possible hazards – I also have to believe he'll ignore all the pizza and chips strewn out along the pavements. Oh, and that he'll remember where to take me back. I can tell you, it'd be a lot better without foodie doggy distractions.

Often I don't feel safe simply because of all the obstacles in our way. Wheelie bins, pushchairs or bicycles are thoughtlessly left out in the middle of the pavement. Imagine what it's like for a sight impaired person negotiating his way round a bike or a pushchair to get into a shop. I've often had to wait outside for someone to come out and move an obstacle so that I can simply get in. If you're one of the culprits maybe you've no idea how frustrating this can be.

Imagine the problems we face...

One of my main bugbears is the way some people behave on the streets. For example, motorists park their cars on the pavement, putting sight impaired people in great danger. Neither long cane users nor guide dog owners can negotiate their way through the narrow gap which results, so they're forced to walk on the road. Not only is this a practical problem, it's also upsetting because pavement parking carries a very clear message: it's basically telling blindies 'Hey! You can't drive, but I can. What's more, I'll park where I like.' While the roads are your means of access, the pavements are ours. And we like to feel we're safe while we're walking on them.

We like to feel safe on the pavements: they're our means of access.

Even town planners wind me up. Street furniture such as waste bins, bollards and benches can be so hazardous. These items need to be very thoughtfully located for the sake of the countless people walking around who can't see as well as they ideally need to. These days town planners even seem to be encouraging cyclists to use pavements or pedestrian zones. More and more often white lines are appearing down the centre of pavements, the idea being that one side should be for pedestrians, the other for cyclists. Have you spotted the problem yet? Yes, you've guessed it: sight impaired people can't see the line so we don't know which side we're supposed to be on or even that there *is* a side we need to be on.

If it's so obvious to you, why can't the idiots at the town hall work it out?

Someone cycling on the pavement at least needs to have the good sense to dismount when he sees a sight impaired person approaching. (It would be better if he could avoid the pavements altogether, of course.) Not only are blindies disorientated by cyclists, guide dogs are too. At best a cyclist can frighten a dog badly. At worst he can ruin its career.

Ordinary residents can also cause enormous problems for people with failing eyesight. If untrimmed trees and bushes overhang a pavement, guide dog owners and long cane users can't find their way forward and they may well sustain unpleasant injuries.

Sight impaired people encounter situations like these on a daily basis. In your own day-to-day life I would hope that you will do what you can to improve the situation because every individual can make a difference. Even if you feel at a loss right now, please don't feel so intimidated and overwhelmed by the problems we face that you end up doing nothing. We need your understanding and support – we really do. If you don't believe me just consider for a moment why it is that according to Guide Dogs for the Blind 180,000 blind and sight impaired people in the UK never go out alone. Nobody helps them gain the skills they need to deal with all these hazards they're likely to encounter, so they simply never build up enough confidence. I know loads of sight impaired people who stay at home all the time and never go out. People like me go out much more, but even then we get scared off every now and then, when we encounter too much stress along the way. A little help from you could make a real difference to so many people's lives.

Chapter 28:

Dog lore

One thing you can certainly do when you're out is approach guide dogs with a helpful and sensitive attitude. It's incredible the number of people who try and talk to Abbot when we're crossing the road. There's actually a school of thought which says you should never talk to a guide dog under any circumstances. This is not something I subscribe to, but I would at least hope you will use your judgment whatever situation you happen to be in. At the very least, make sure you never distract a guide dog while he's working.

Actually, there's an even better approach than that... *Before* you make any move towards a guide dog, make contact with its owner first. Of course, you shouldn't attempt this until you're sure the guide dog owner is in a place of safety. Then, you might ask if it's OK to fuss their dog. When you do this, remember that there might be a vital reason why the owner doesn't want you fussing their dog at that particular time. It may be that the dog is somewhat distracted at the time and fussing may cause the dog to become overexcited. Or the reason may be much more mundane: maybe the owner is simply running late and you have not been the first one to ask to fuss the dog on this particular journey. After all, these are very popular dogs.

A simple trip to the local shop which may take a sighted person ten minutes can take me twice as long simply because of the number of people who want to make a fuss of Abbot. Sometimes this is fine and no one enjoys it more than me. Then there are days when time is at a premium and I need to press on. There have been several occasions when people's feelings have been hurt because I didn't have time for them to fuss over Abbot.

The next rule is never to grab a guide dog's harness. The harness is a sensitive instrument and needs to be treated with respect. If you should happen to see a guide dog owner standing still with his dog's harness laid flat on the dog's back this may be a sign that he's in difficulty. It may be a good idea to offer to help. Guide dog owners often carry a little sign with the word 'HELP' on it. If ever you see one of us holding up such a sign, please do help.

Never grab a guide dog's harness.

Beyond this, whenever you speak to a guide dog owner about his dog, do please remember that he may feel very sensitive about any negative comments. Denise and I don't have any children and have not experienced the joy or pain of parenthood. However, I have caught myself being an over-protective parent from time to time. Occasionally, someone will pass a seemingly innocent remark about Abbot which I will interpret as a criticism. If this person says something like 'He's a big lad' I immediately get all defensive and start thinking negative things to myself. (So do they mean he's not the correct weight? Are they saying he's fat? Would they like a smack in the mouth?) It might be easier for you to understand this if you remember that Abbot and me are really a single unit... so if you pick on him, you pick on me. Perhaps this is why, when someone asks me if Abbot bites I say:

"No, he doesn't. But I might."

Actually, it's very unlikely that anyone could legitimately criticise Abbot because of his weight. As his owner I'm the person who's responsible for feeding him. Abbot is on Eukanuba, which is a dried food. He gets a total of 350 grams per day, half in the morning and half in the evening. He's fed to a whistle, so as to make sure there's a sound that can be made to call him back, if ever that's necessary. For this reason, whenever Abbot is out for a free run I always carry a small biscuit in my pocket. Then I just blow my whistle when I want him to return and give him the biscuit. After all these years it's deeply engrained in Abbot that the sound of his whistle equals food. This is because each time I feed him, morning and evening, I place his bowl of food on the floor and tell him to wait. He can only eat when I blow his whistle and give him the command 'Take it'. I strive to keep Abbot's mealtimes to the same time each day, although this is not always possible. Keeping him to regular mealtimes means that he also has regular spending times, which means that I can arrange my day around those times.

Within this routine, titbits are definitely not allowed, as I've explained already. Guide Dogs set a maximum weight for each dog and dogs are weighed every six months. If a dog weighs over his maximum weight three times in a row he is removed from service, so you can see how important it is that he isn't fed between meals. Abbot is a typical labrador – a life support system for a stomach – so his weight needs constant watching. Other people often accuse me of being cruel because I'm so strict about his diet but it's vital that he maintain a healthy weight since lab retrievers are particularly prone to many weight-related health problems.

If ever Abbot does develop a health problem, it is again my responsibility to take him to the vet and then if necessary, administer any medication. In the last few months Abbot has been suffering from a very persistent ear infection. I have spent many a hilarious evening chasing him round the kitchen with a ball of cotton wool and some ointment.

Grooming is also a very important part of the care I'm required to take over Abbot – so again, criticising him for the way he looks is very much like criticising me. Every time we go out Abbot must be groomed because this is part of the legal contract I have with Guide Dogs.

First he has to be rubbed down with a chamois leather (a shammy). Then I groom him with a tool called a 'Zoom Groom', which is a type of rubber brush. And finally I comb him. (This process takes about 15-20 minutes.) Some days Abbot and I go out more than once and this process has to be repeated each time. Often we set off with Abbot looking better turned out than his owner! If Abbot goes in the sea or becomes muddy then of course he must be given a bath. Bathing and grooming are the sole responsibility of the owner. This is to assist in the bonding process between dog and owner. People who can't commit to doing this simply aren't given a guide dog.

'Spending' Abbot (i.e. getting him to wee and poo) is again my responsibility and spending other than at home is not encouraged unless under extreme circumstances. (In any case guide dogs are not allowed to foul in the street.) Of course it's also my job to bag and pick up. Not doing so is again an offence that can result in a dog being removed.

If ever you encounter a guide dog owner whose dog is not obeying any of these rules, you can be sure he or she is in breach of his contract with Guide Dogs. (It's very unlikely, of course, because that would mean the guide dog would be taken away from its owner.)

Generally, we guide dog owners have to be a very well-disciplined bunch of people.

Generally, we guide dog owners have to be a very well-disciplined bunch of people. And most of us realise that we're also ambassadors for the Guide Dogs for the Blind organisation. For this reason, it's unlikely you'll meet an owner who's rude to you if you try to approach their dog (after asking, of course). If you do – and I have heard a few rather nasty stories, I must admit – please accept my apologies on behalf of any grumpy guide dog owner. Perhaps they're having a bad day and they've ended up snapping at you after enduring abuse from countless other people before you...

Chapter 29:

Before Abbot

In case you're wondering why I go to all this trouble so as to have a guide dog, let me explain what a difference it makes to me. Here's a typical day as it was before I got Abbot. I'm going to describe a trip into Newcastle as it used to be.

Walking up my street isn't too bad because I'm in familiar surroundings. However, when someone steps out of their garden gate I crash into them. This is quite simply because they've come from outside the bounds of my limited peripheral vision and I don't see them until it's too late. They call me an idiot. Moving on up the street someone opens their car door and again it's outside my peripheral vision so I walk into it. I apologise but as I walk away I'm sure I can hear someone mutter the word 'idiot' again.

Feeling more than a little hurt I make it to the top of the street without further incident. I'm now walking alongside the main Newcastle road. The traffic is very busy and I'm feeling more than a little intimidated. No one seems to be sticking to the 30 mph speed limit and I can feel the tension beginning to rise within me. Before crossing the road I decide to go into the newsagent's to buy a lottery ticket. The slip that you fill in is too small for me to read so I ask the man behind the counter if he'd mind filling it in for me. He snatches it from me and grudgingly fills it in, muttering something about me being a bit thick. I'm beginning to think about calling off my trip to save myself any further humiliation.

Leaving the newsagent's, I head for the zebra crossing so as to get across that busy Newcastle road. A car is approaching the crossing but I can't judge his speed so I wait at the kerb until he's completely stopped. The driver is already impatient that I haven't set off over the crossing as he approached and he's now revving his engine. I can feel myself getting more and more uptight. As I pass his windscreen he's tapping his head with his index finger, indicating that I'm an idiot.

I manage to make it safely to the bus stop. After a while I can see something that looks like it might be a bus. It's big and red so maybe it's a fire engine. (I have been known to flag them down in the past. I once flagged down a cement mixer.) As the big red vehicle gets closer I realise it really is a bus so I stick my hand out. I can't read the number while the bus is moving so I have to flag him anyway. As soon as he's stopped the driver opens the door and I ask him if he's the 527. His reply is 'Are you fucking blind or what?' As he shuts the door he calls me a 'fucking idiot'. I'm on the verge of going home, I feel so demoralised. This was supposed to be an enjoyable shopping trip but it's turning into a nightmare of ridicule and abuse.

The next bus to arrive is mine and I manage to make it safely on board. After a short journey I leave the bus to make the rest of the journey by Metro. In case you're wondering how I know when to get off, it's actually quite simple. With my level of sight I can easily recognise the eight-foot-high, illuminated sign at Heworth Metro station. Getting through the station and finding the platform is not too difficult but on the platform there's a moving digital display which I simply cannot read.

As a train approaches I ask the man next to me if this is the train for Newcastle. He just points at the digital display and walks off.

"Thanks for all your help," I say. And he walks off muttering abuse.

Fortunately, it is in fact the right train and I make it safely into Newcastle. On leaving the train at Newcastle I have to pass through a turnstile. It's very busy and there are people coming at me from both sides from beyond the bounds of my peripheral vision. I can't help but bump into one of them and once again a total stranger calls me an idiot. I can feel my temper starting to go.

Now I'm making my way up Northumberland Street, the main shopping street in Newcastle. This is a pedestrian zone with shops on both sides. People are emerging from shop doorways on both sides of the street but because of my lack of peripheral vision I'm simply not picking up on them and I'm bumping into them constantly. 'Idiot,' they all mutter. By now my temper is completely out of the bag.

I've heard on the radio that there's a new Jackson Browne CD out so I wander into HMV. The shop is badly lit and once again I'm bumping into people. The combination of bad lighting and the small print on CD covers make it impossible for me to find what I'm looking for so I go off in search of an assistant. Eventually, I track one down and she tells me that if they have what I want it'll be out there on the shelves and that I should go and look. I'm almost at boiling point now and I'm forcing my hands into my pockets to avoid choking the assistant. I skulk out of the store feeling embarrassed and defeated.

Comfort for such feelings comes in the form of a burger. So off I set in search of a fast-food joint. The menus in such establishments are always situated high up on a back wall, behind the counter. It's impossible for me to read the list of food items so I ask the 18-year-old behind the counter what they have. She points at the sign and says:

"Duh, it's up there."

I've had more than enough for one day.

The red mist has now completely descended and I've had more than enough for one day. I swear at the child behind the counter and storm out of the store. Sod it. I'm going home, I think to myself. Just then I bump into another man who's come up on my blind side. His meal is now spread all down his shirt and he's not looking too happy.

"IDIOT!" he shouts.

"Fuck off," I reply as I bolt for the Metro station.

The return journey is just as fraught as the outward one but by now the pan of my temper has completely boiled over.

Before Abbot came along there were many days like this and I had simply stopped going out on my own altogether. I would ask other people to go shopping for me and I avoided socialising on my own. By the time Abbot came along, apart from hospital appointments it had been over 18 months since I'd been out alone.

Chapter 30:

With Abbot

Here's a retake of the last chapter. This time I have the services of a guide dog.

When Abbot and I are all groomed and ready – or at least, when Abbot is – we set off. Abbot's in the lead, wearing a white harness (as opposed to a brown one), which proves that he's fully qualified as a guide dog. I'm following behind, sensitive to Abbot's every movement.

Moving beyond the familiar terrain of the garden and the gate, we proceed up the street. Suddenly, I feel Abbot's harness move to the left and I move with it. This is now second nature to me. It isn't until we pass that I realise a man was coming out of his gate and we have missed him completely. I bump into no one and no one calls me an idiot. Marvellous, bloody marvellous.

We turn right and walk along that busy Newcastle road. The fast-moving traffic holds no terror for me now. I utter that magic key word 'News' and Abbot heads for the newsagent's. As we enter, the man behind the counter shouts,

"Hi, Dave! How's Abbot?"

I give him my lottery ticket and he fills it out for me and we exchange some friendly banter. Once again, no one has called me an idiot.

Coming out I use another one of those key words 'Crossing' and Abbot takes me to the zebra crossing. We wait at the kerb for a few moments until the traffic comes to a stop. I give Abbot the command 'Forward' and Abbot heads purposefully across the road.

As we go past one of the waiting cars I think I can see one of the drivers smiling and pointing at Abbot. Marvellous, bloody marvellous.

We make it safely to the bus stop and wait a few moments for the bus to arrive. When it does, the doors open and the driver calls out the number asking if this is the one I need. As it happens this is not the one for me but I thank him anyway and he tells me that the one I want will be along shortly. Sure enough my bus is right behind and we make it safely on board.

On arrival at the Metro station we make it safely to the platform. As we're waiting a gentleman asks us what train we're waiting for. He assures me the next train is for Newcastle and asks if I mind if he pats my dog. He's been so helpful, I'm only too pleased to let him.

As we board the train and I sit down Abbot begins to play his favourite game. He sits between my feet, head resting on my knee, looking as pathetic as possible. He scans the carriage to see who's taking notice of him. When he finds his victim he fixes them with his most soulful expression. His face asks the question: 'Would you like to give me a pat?' In my experience there are few people who can resist this and you can bet your bottom dollar that within a few moments his chosen victim will cave in and come over and ask if he can give him a pat. It never fails and Abbot, the celebrity, has another adoring fan. Bless him.

We alight in Newcastle city centre and as we progress through the turnstile I begin to realise that no one has bumped into me even though there are people coming at me from all sides. Abbot is very much in control in these situations and it's now a matter of habit for me to tune into the movement of his harness and to move with it, thus avoiding physical contact with any passers by. We are now on Northumberland Street and although people are coming out of shop doorways from outside my visual field, I haven't as much as brushed sleeves with anyone. This is what Abbot lives for. His tail is up and he's giving it 100% concentration and taking great pride in his work. For the first time in years I'm enjoying a shopping trip. I haven't made physical contact with anyone and no one has called me an idiot or abused me in any other way. This is such a joy.

I decide to try my luck at finding that Jackson Browne CD again. So off I set for HMV. As I walk into the shop a shop assistant spots us and asks if she can be of any help. I tell her what I'm looking for and she tells me to wait where I am and she goes away to find it for me. I can't believe it! There's been no need for me to go through the embarrassment of telling a total stranger about my sight impairment. Wow! I stand waiting, feeling appreciative of Abbot. By now I'm getting a little big-headed and I'm beginning to think I've got this whole shopping thing in the bag. Feeling more than a little pleased with myself, I decide to have another go at sampling burger cuisine. I join the queue and await the attention of the 18-year-old behind the counter. I ask her if she can tell me what's on the menu.

"It's on the board up there," she mutters.

I'm standing in front of her wearing dark glasses, carrying a symbol cane and I've got Abbot in full working harness, complete with fluorescent markings. Obviously both her neurons are out to lunch. She points again at the board and mumbles: "Up there."

At this point she's very close to serious harm. I am about to unleash the wrath that has been building up in me over 30 years. Suddenly, I feel a tugging at my sleeve and I turn to find a very petite lady standing beside me.

I am about to unleash the wrath of 30 years...

"WHAT?!" Addressing her, I completely forget I'm no longer talking to the thicko 18-year-old behind the counter.

"I thought you might like me to read the menu to you," she begins nervously.

This is another of those 'Oh bugger' moments. I've allowed my temper to trample all over the feelings of a lovely lady who is simply trying to help. I apologise profusely and she tells me she understands perfectly. She sits beside me as I settle down at a table and Abbot crawls underneath. As I munch happily on my burger she fusses over Abbot and becomes yet another fully signed-up member of the Abbot Fan Club. Membership must by now outnumber that of Robbie Williams' and Abbot doesn't even have a tattoo. He doesn't wear an earring and the only drugs he does are his anti-flea treatment.

So you see... Life *with* Abbot is a whole lot better than life *before* Abbot. He's a wonderful being and his talents are the stuff of legend. Nevertheless, having given you a glimpse into my 'before' and 'after' worlds I don't want to give you the impression that a guide dog is the cure-all for every issue of sight impairment. The world has more than its fair share of people who are ignorant of the issues involved in sight impairment. More on that later...

Chapter 31:

Out on the town

More than anything, Abbot has given me back a social life. Evenings were always my worst time of day as both darkness and tiredness affect my sight. Even now I'm at my least confident when it gets dark as I'm totally night blind. But I do go out now... That's quite simply because Abbot is like a beacon that lights up even the darkest night. This means that evenings and nights no longer hold any terror so now that I'm in my late 40s I have a better social life than I ever did in my early 20s.

And of course Abbot is a star at all my regular haunts. (Denise has even been heard to complain about this, but we both know she wouldn't change things for the world.) If I book tickets for a concert at the Tyne Theatre they always ask if Abbot is coming so they can have a bowl of water and a red carpet at the ready. Abbot has been to several performances where he's upstaged the main act.

I was late booking my tickets for the Richard Thompson concert last year. The only seats they had left were way up in the gods. I knew there was no room for Abbot up there so my friend George came along as my sighted guide. As we entered the foyer the manageress spotted us and asked where Abbot was. I explained the situation and she moved two journalists out of the front row so we had a better view. George was highly impressed and is thinking of getting a guide dog of his own. There's nothing wrong with his sight – he just likes the perks that go with it.

I told you that hanging around with celebrities has a certain kudos. When we visit my local pub, usually on a Friday evening, the barman refuses to let anyone sit in Abbot's place. Abbot had only been around for a few weeks when they presented him with his own water bowl with his name on. They watch for us coming past the window and by the time we get to the bar they have his bowl of water ready for him. Me, I have to queue up for my drink like everyone else.

Abbot has so many fans in the pub that if I miss a Friday for any reason, they hold an inquest. When I was ill they all offered to collect Abbot and take him to the pub so they could still have their Friday night with him. There's a group of rugby players, all big lads, and they've adopted Abbot as their own. Woe betide anyone who upsets him. Someone tried to sit in Abbot's spot one evening and before I could do anything, this person had been threatened with violence. The poor guy left without a word and has not been seen since.

Given this level of personal support, which I get when people get to know me and Abbot, I really wonder why there isn't more generalised support. I mean, why won't people help us unless they get to know us? The main problem, I think, is that society has changed so much over the last few decades and not always for the better.

As a young man I was very lucky. I didn't know it then but in hindsight I realise I was very blessed. I was surrounded by people who had a strong sense of social justice. There was my grandmother, Father Bill Rooke (a local priest), my friend Leo and also countless others who showed me that we have a duty to those less fortunate. They taught me that we must carry people who are not able to walk alone – not literally, you'll be pleased to hear! – until such time that they can stand on their own, if ever that day comes. These good folk, who were my role models, would give until it hurt and then carry on and give some more.

As society becomes more apathetic and more secular we're in danger of losing educators who will instil these qualities in the young. Governments have tried to compensate for this by legislation and this is great but it also reflects a sad state of affairs. After all, it's difficult to legislate for what is essentially a matter of conscience. Conscience must be learned by example and, sadly, there are fewer and fewer people these days setting a positive example.

Experts on disability imply there are two ways of viewing sight impairment: the medical model and the social model. In the medical model the person with failing eyesight is seen as a problem – he can't see, he may be housebound, he may have difficulty with stairs, he may need help with a carer and, to make matters worse, he may also be looking for a cure. Within the social model, on the other hand, the *world* is seen as the problem – buildings are not designed well, transport is inaccessible to too many people, there's a lack of information, people are prejudiced, education is segregated, jobs are not open to all and some families remain isolated.

Since the law in the UK is based on the medical model, the relevant law – the Disability Discrimination Act (DDA) – depends on concepts such as 'reasonable adjustment' and 'minimum standards' to meet the needs of disabled people. And the money needed to make even these so-called 'reasonable' adjustments is all-too-often not made available. To make matters worse, nobody is policed, legal action is rarely possible when individuals or organisations break the law (again, for financial reasons), and charities which support the needs of sight impaired people receive no government funding.

> With a complete lack of government funding we don't seem to be making much progress in terms of making positive change.

With this medical model and a complete lack of government funding we certainly don't seem to be making much progress in terms of making positive change.

Chapter 32:

Show us your money

Ever since I got Abbot I've wanted to do something to help other people with sight impairment. As a result, I now wear many hats within Guide Dogs and dedicate a great deal of time to the charity. Abbot and I can be seen all over the region and beyond, most weekends and many evenings. The more guide dog owners who get involved in this way, the better. Working alongside sighted people, we really will be able to change things for the better.

> Working alongside sighted people we really will be able to change things for the better.

Four years ago my friend Dave Newton and I embarked on a project to make a film about Guide Dogs and some of the issues faced by sight impaired people. We decided to call the film *The Road Ahead* and to form a trust called Road Ahead in order to raise the necessary funding. Road Ahead has grown and grown and we have now made other films and organised concerts on behalf of Guide Dogs too. (These now seem to have become annual events.) We have also taken over the running of an annual carol service for Guide Dogs, performing the music, publishing the song book in various formats and putting on a do afterwards. As for the original film, *The Road Ahead*, it's been seen by many audiences, many copies have been sold and many other doors have opened to us because of that one little film. Of course, it's also raised a lot of money for Guide Dogs.

I've also spearheaded a few other fundraising activities. In 2002 we arranged a Christmas carol service at Sunderland Minster. The church was full of dogs: working guide dogs and their owners, guide dog puppies and their puppy walkers, retired guide dogs and their carers. We even had dogs that hadn't quite made it as guide dogs, who'd come along with their proud new owners. (Guide Dogs refer to such dogs as 'rejects', which is not a term I like. It seems to suggest the dog is inferior in some way. I like to think they simply have a different skill set.) Anyway, here we were with all these dogs and there was no fighting. Well, not amongst the dogs anyway.

I'd been asked to give a reading and had been allocated a seat near the front. I had just made myself comfortable when I felt a tap on my shoulder and turned to find Ken, one of my trainers, sitting behind me. He remarked that Abbot and I looked great together and asked if I remembered what he'd told me, that it takes roughly a year to form a good partnership. It was almost a year to the day since Abbot and I qualified.

"You should see us working together now," I said. "He's an absolute star!"

"I have," he replied. "I've just followed you all the way through Sunderland." He always was a sneaky sod.

Canon Bryan Hales, a great friend to Guide Dogs, walked up to the lectern.

"I have some notices," he said. Usually church notices talk about the next meeting of the Parish Council or the WI or when the Sunday school outing will be. Not these ones...

"Poop bags are available in the narthex," he began.

A smile was spreading across my face. "There are water bowls at intervals down the aisles and – should your dog need to spend a penny – there's a designated spending area in the churchyard." Before Brian could finish speaking the tears were streaming down my face and I was chewing the back of my hand in a vain attempt to smother my laughter. Denise was digging me in the ribs, telling me it wasn't funny, but we both knew it was hilarious. Other people were beginning to stare and Ken was punching me in the back telling me to stop – before I set him off too. Throughout the service I would periodically remember that little list of notices and would have to compose myself all over again.

Apart from that little blip, it was a great service. We had sight impaired readers and musicians and the atmosphere was terrific. The church was filled with a wonderful atmosphere that made the hairs on the back of my neck stand on end, just like that first time at the Guide Dog Centre. So inspired was I that for the last four years I've put together a growing band of musicians to lead the music at what is now an annual carol service.

There was a wonderful atmosphere.

Then in January 2004 something particularly wonderful happened involving Allan Taylor, the singer- songwriter I mentioned earlier, who's been a hero of mine since I was 17 (over 30 years ago). He seemed so much older than me when I was a teenager, so that must make him about 99 now. And yet he still looks younger than me. More importantly, he still plays the guitar so much better than me.

More than any other songwriter, Allan's songs have seen me through many dark days and have played a part in many important parts of my life. For example, Denise and I had someone perform a dance to Allan's song 'Now You Know' at our wedding. I can pinpoint significant points in my life by the song of Allan's that meant most to me at that time. At 17 all I wanted to do was *be* Allan Taylor, but sadly I was never going to be good enough. Allan's guitar sound was such an inspiration, though, that I spent ages saving up to buy my first Martin guitar. I've owned a few Martins since... I have one now but I still can't make it sound like Allan's. Just recently Allan came to my home and he played my Martin. It sounded bloody great. Why doesn't it sound like that when I play it?

Allan travels all over the world performing and is seldom at home long enough to get involved in fundraising events, but when I asked if he'd do a gig for Guide Dogs he didn't hesitate. Local comedy duo Maxi and Mitch, who are mates of mine, are also old friends of Allan's so Allan suggested I ask them to take part too. They also readily agreed.

You can't imagine what a coup this was for me. To have Allan come and play would have been more than enough, but to have the added bonus of Maxi and Mitch was wonderful. I would dine out on this for quite some time to come. It was a great night and we raised a lot of money. Allan began his set with what is perhaps his best known song, a song called 'It's Good To See You'. A ripple of nervous laughter rang round the room (get it?) and it took a while for Allan to realise his mistake. Although some of us couldn't in fact see him we could feel the glow from his embarrassed face right at the back of the room.

Of course, this was just an obvious thing to say and it's not even offensive to people with a sight impairment. After all, it's just part of our language, isn't it?

Nevertheless, Maxi and Mitch milked this heavily during their act afterwards. I've attended many of Allan's concerts since then with my friend Alex (who is also blind) and we've started a tradition of waving our white canes in the air when Allan gets to the chorus of this song. It's like being at a Barry Manilow concert when people wave their lighters in the air. Mind you, to be fair to Allan, his nose is not as big as Barry's.

We've started a tradition of waving our white canes in the air during the chorus.

There have also been other fundraising events: four concerts in all and more are being planned. Also, I give talks about Guide Dogs and hardly a week goes by when my puppy-walking friend, Ethne Brown, and I aren't out giving a talk. I'm the volunteer liaison officer for our region and the list of activities I'm involved in is endless.

However, although all this fundraising activity is enjoyable, I have to ask why it's necessary at all. If I had any other illness or disability that required a mobility aid such as a wheelchair or stairlift it would be provided by the NHS. Why should it be any different for a person needing a guide dog?

Chapter 33:

You think I can't do it?

A couple of years ago, on the run up to Denise's birthday I was talking to a friend about what I might get her as a present. While we were talking, this friend doubted that I'd be able to do the shopping myself (forgetting Abbot, of course) and suggested I get someone else to do my shopping for me. He told me it was a long time since I'd been into town on my own and that my sight had deteriorated since then.

It was perfectly true I hadn't been into town *on my own* for a long time, but for some reason hearing this seemed to get right under my skin. I felt more riled than I would have thought possible – somehow backed into a corner. The old Dave took over and I suddenly heard myself boasting that I could get into town and do my shopping without Abbot, or anyone else's help for that matter. You know how it is? You just know it's going to end in tears but there's no fool like an old fool.

Isn't it strange how when you know you're about to do something stupid you can come up with all kinds of justification? I told myself that my hands would be full of shopping and I'd therefore be unable to work Abbot in any case. How could there be a problem? Only a few years earlier, before Abbot, I'd been going into town on my own fairly regularly. Things couldn't have changed that much. I was like a child who'd been given a dare: there was serious pride at stake. I would do it even if it killed me! With the state of my sight these days, that was a very strong possibility.

Off I set. I made my way down the first road. Then, by standing at the zebra crossing with a bunch of other pedestrians and crossing when they did, I made it across the main road. I was beginning to feel very smug indeed. Well, as you know, pride comes before a fall and mine was just around the corner. I arrived at the top of the stairs that lead down to my local Metro train station. These stairs are very steep and appear to me to be almost a vertical drop. I didn't so much as descend the stairs as throw myself off the top. More by luck than good judgement I arrived unscathed at the bottom, but I was feeling more than a little shaken. As I moved towards the platform that shaky feeling returned and I became convinced I would fall onto the track. I moved back against the wall and clung to it until the train arrived.

Once on board, I had time to realise that my sight had got a lot worse since the last time I'd done this. I realised I'd come to rely on Abbot to do all the concentrating for me. All the danger and stress of being a sight impaired person out alone came flooding back. However, I was still determined to go through with my self-imposed challenge. After all, a dare is a dare and I was going to show them, wasn't I?

By the time I got into central Newcastle I was in total panic. I bumped into dozens of people coming out of the Metro and most of them showered abuse on my head. As I stepped out of the underground station into the daylight the sudden change in light level was too much. The bit of sight I normally have was temporarily wiped out and I couldn't see anything at all.

The bit of sight I normally have was wiped out.

I groped my way to a bench and had to sit for quite some time till my eyes adjusted. I headed straight back home in a taxi to pick up Abbot. We headed back into town together and everything was fine.

So I've learned my lesson: where I go, Abbot goes too. We two are one. We're a team, a true partnership. Abbot is always ready to help, if only I'll let him. Sometimes, though, I have to admit, this 'help' was not all selfless in the early days. I suppose this may go some way to explaining why I still wanted to regress to my earlier so-called independence around that time. Lynne, Abbot's trainer, has now cured Abbot of all his early problems but you might be interested to hear that it wasn't all plain sailing at first. In those early days I wasn't the only one who had some lessons to learn.

For example, one day quite early on Abbot and I were walking along towards a bus stop. A bus happened to pull up just at that point and Abbot tried to take me on board. I wouldn't have minded, but I wasn't going that way on that particular day... Another 'problem' we had at first involved our local butcher's shop. Twice one week I'd been picked up opposite this shop and each time, while we were waiting for our lift, Jim (the butcher) had come over to make a fuss of Abbot. Of course, as we waited in the same spot on the third day, which happened to be a Sunday, Abbot fixed the butcher's window with a purposeful stare.

"He's not there today," I said, but Abbot showed his frustration by stamping his paws as he let out an enormous 'WOOF!' Fortunately, Jim arrived at this point and further tantrums were avoided.

Another time, a hailstorm started while Abbot and I were travelling into Gateshead by taxi. When we reached our destination, Abbot took one look out the window and refused point blank to leave the taxi. The taxi driver roared with laughter and was more than happy for Abbot to sit there until the storm had passed.

Abbot refused point blank to leave the taxi.

As I said, Abbot has now been cured of these early problems, just as I've learned my lesson about going out alone. I do still miss being able to go out on my own, I must admit. Being out without a dog was more discreet – I didn't feel as 'on show' and self-conscious. I know those days are over but I still grieve for my independence and the wound is not properly healed. Nevertheless, being Abbot's dad has its own reward. Abbot is my boy and I'm his dad and like any proud father I love to show him off.

Chapter 34:

He can see, you know

When I first got Abbot I was registered sight impaired but such is the rate of deterioration that I was registered blind in 2004. (Now there is no longer a category 'blind' – it's 'severely sight impaired'.) Even though I am registered blind (or 'severely sight impaired') I still have some useful sight in my right eye. This is a concept that many of the public have difficulty with. Some folk would rather I pretend I can see nothing at all than deal with the idea that someone with a long cane or guide dog has some useful sight. But let's be reasonable here: you wouldn't insist that a person who'd lost a leg should have the other leg removed before he could be defined as a cripple, would you?

Sight impaired people need to be treated with respect and allowed to make the best of what useful vision remains. However, some people seem to disagree... Total strangers demand detailed explanations of my medical history and feel they have a right to know. Imagine what that's like. Someone you've never met before stops you in the street and asks you if you have piles and, if so, how they affect your life. Then they go on to ask if they can take a look. This is the kind of thing that happens to me all the time. I have stood at a bus stop while a woman has circled all the way round me waving her hands in the air to see if I could see her. People come up really close and stick up fingers so that I can tell them how many. They pull faces and stick their tongues out at me and if I react they're convinced I'm a fake – not a real blindy at all.

Sight impaired people are subjected to this kind of questioning – or should I say abuse? – on a daily basis. But it's precisely this kind of behaviour that drives sight impaired people onto the offensive and it may cause them to snap at the very next person that approaches them.

There are some people out there who think I only got Abbot to strengthen my case with the benefits agency. Let me tell you that the pitiful amount I get is not enough to compensate for the amount of abuse I get from the public. I can think of other ways to scam the benefits agency that do not involve daily humiliation.

In the days before Abbot, when I bumped into someone I was usually greeted with the words 'Are you fucking blind or what?!'

Now the same people mutter 'He can see, you know!' There are days when I feel confident and empowered and I can rise above such things. Then there are the black days when I feel like a freak show exhibit and I want to run for home, lock the door and never go out again. People point as I pass by. They pass comment without even affording me the courtesy of lowering their voice. Some days, if I'm walking along with Denise, I promise her the next person who annoys me will suffer my anger. This usually turns out to be the one person who is trying to help. You have no idea how many shopping trips have ended with Denise and me having a huge row over the way I've spoken to someone.

There are black days when I feel like a freak show exhibit and want to run for home.

I was in my local pub one night when a complete stranger sat himself right in front of me at my table and began waving his hand in front of my face. I didn't react immediately but when he continued to persist I grabbed his wrist. He turned to his mates crying 'I told you he could see!' My rugby-playing friends took him outside for a quiet word and frankly I'm not at all bothered.

My rugby-playing friends took him outside...

This type of behaviour is just so hurtful. It's what causes some sight impaired people to withdraw from society altogether. I refuse to be driven to this but I do have bad days. Days when for an instant I regret going on the register and getting a guide dog. But then Abbot sticks his head up for a pat and I know I wouldn't change a thing, not for any money. If it wasn't for Abbot I'd have dropped out of society by now. It's not my self confidence that keeps me going, it's the love I get from Abbot and his faith in me.

For me being sight impaired is in some ways like being a recovering alcoholic. Every morning I wake up and recommit myself to another day as a sight impaired person. 'Hello, everyone. My name is Dave and I'm severely sight impaired.' There are days when I regret my decision both to register as sight impaired and also to get Abbot. If I didn't have such a strong bond with Abbot I may have given up by now. It isn't my self-confidence that keeps me going, it's my belief in Abbot.

Chapter 35:

Flashback

February 5th

It's almost midnight and I'm reflecting on a day that I've feared all my life. Today my consultant told me it was time to change my registration status from visually impaired to blind. Years ago I was so gripped with fear at this prospect I would just have run and cursed the world at the injustice of it all. I always thought that this moment would be too much to cope with... Yet here it is and while it's not good news, it doesn't scare me anything like I thought it would. My vision is failing and I may not keep even the sight I have now but I have Abbot in my life so it feels like anything is possible. His belief in me is awe-inspiring and life is good. Abbot sees enough for both of us. This last year has been the happiest time in my life and what happened today is a mere blip on life's radar. The world has not fallen apart as I always thought it might. The old feeling of 'Let's run!' has not surfaced. I have a strong feeling that we are now into uncharted territory. Just as I wrote that, Abbot wandered into the room and sat down beside me as if to say 'It'll be OK, Dad.' And do you know what? I think he might just be right. Now I really am a true blindy and I don't give a stuff. I love Denise, she loves me and Abbot and Tessa love us both. What more is there? Good night and God bless. (Bloody hell, this diary is starting to sound like *The Waltons*.)

I'm a true blindy and I don't give a stuff.

February 10th

These are strange days indeed. Since last week's news I find myself looking at familiar things in a new light. I watch Denise as she's sleeping and try and freeze the picture in my memory. I want to hold such pictures in my mind forever. Now and again I'm consumed by the fear that I might not be able to remember. Now and again I'm seized by the enormity of it all. I've never known fear like this.

February 14th

The practicalities of my sight loss are not the things that frighten me. Abbot has taught me that all such things are surmountable. No, it's a grieving process for all the familiar things that I know I'll miss terribly.

February 18th

Every time I look at someone or something that's important to me, I find myself wondering if this is the last time I'll see that particular scene. I try and force such images into some kind of mental filing cabinet in the vain hope that I might be able to call them up at some point in the dreadful, sightless future.

February 21st

I'm more confident in Abbot's powers than at any time since his arrival. I know that in a practical sense we will cope admirably. But like a child reading in bed I keep bargaining with God to leave the light on for just five more minutes. Please, God. Just five more minutes.

Deep in my heart I know we'll be OK.

February 22nd

Abbot's my rock and deep in my heart I know we'll be OK but right now I feel so lost and all at sea.

February 24th

There is no handbook for where I'm at now and this is so much a period of learning. I've no way of knowing if I'm handling things the right way. All I know is that with Abbot's help I'm getting through it and although it may not be pretty to watch, we're far from beaten. I've still got my independence. Abbot is helping me keep my dignity, which is the most important thing.

February 26th

The panic I've felt in recent days still rears its ugly head from time to time but I'll be damned if I'll let it win. I know now just how far we've come and I'm not going to give up now. In Abbot's head we two are one and in the last few days he's assumed a new responsibility for my well-being. I'm not facing this alone. Abbot is right here in the midst of it all, constantly checking to see if I'm OK.

> The panic I've felt in recent days still rears its ugly head from time to time but I'll be damned if I'll let it win.

March 10th

Today is my 44th birthday and it's now over a month since I got the bad news from my consultant. Days like this are landmarks. It's time to take stock. This last month has been an emotional roller coaster. There have been days full of optimism and hope and then black days when I feel the whole world can fuck off. But I'm still here and the panic is subsiding. This is Dave-plus-Abbot. Nothing is impossible. I've placed all my faith in Abbot and he'll get me through this period. He's never let me down so far. He's counting on me as much as I'm counting on him and I can't let him down. We're partners to the end.

He's counting on me as much as I'm counting on him and I can't let him down.

Chapter 36:

Progress?

Actually, my frustration about society's reactions to blind people goes some way to explaining why I put off registering as sight impaired for so long. I was convinced that services for sight impaired people were stuck in the 1950s.

Various professionals tried to change my mind and I discovered that, yes, things have changed since my '60s childhood, but only a little. For example, when my eyesight deteriorated to the extent that I was forced to leave my job in bakery management (way back in 1987, when I was just 27) I went along to my local Job Centre. I explained to the Disability Officer there that my sight impairment meant I could no longer drive or be around heavy equipment, both of which were essential parts of my job, and I also showed him my CV. He said he could arrange a place for me at a skill centre where I would learn to make coat hangers. Can you imagine how thrilling this seemed after bakery management? Not only would it mean a complete lifestyle change it would also mean an incredible fall from grace in terms of finance and status.

When I tried to get some more information about my personal situation and possibilities for my future, I encountered another problem. I was visiting a local society and was perusing a stand full of literature given to the society by the RNIB. Among these leaflets I came across one on nystagmus, one of my conditions. I was about to help myself to a copy when the lady at reception asked my address. When I told her she informed me that I lived outside their catchment area and took the free leaflet off me.

A couple of years later, soon after getting Abbot, I was attending a workshop on blindness when I realised it was the very same lady giving the keynote speech. Her opening line was about the need to supply more sight impaired people with free information on their eye condition. She could see me laughing and suddenly the penny dropped...

Suddenly the penny dropped...

Things improved a little for people with sight impairment when the Disability Discrimination Act (DDA) was passed in 1995 and amended in 2005. The introduction of Disability Equality Duty was also a step forward since it theoretically gave new rights to people with sight impairment. (This came into force in December 2006 with the aim of ensuring that public bodies pay 'due regard' to the promotion of equality for disabled people in every area of their work.)

The only problem is that while passing these acts no one allocated any extra resources so as to make them a reality. This means that many facilities which should be provided under DDA are still not in place. It also means that organisations for the sight impaired lack the resources to bring to account those who are failing to provide good service to sight impaired people. And ironically, for financial reasons, it's often the organisations which represent the sight impaired that fail to implement policies and procedures that comply with DDA.

No one provided any extra resources.

No test cases are brought forward.

We therefore have laws in place but no resources available to the bodies that should represent and defend the interests of sight impaired people – so no test cases are brought forward. There is even a great reluctance to facilitate test cases because doing so would be seen as a political act and might be unattractive to potential funders. I can understand the predicament but this hesitancy means that people who are having difficulty with their eyesight are being denied their rights and no one is standing up for them.

Eventually, after registering as sight impaired and joining that particular 'club' within society, I became absolutely incensed when I heard about an initiative launched by central government a couple of years ago and later farmed out to local authorities. The initiative was called 'Supporting People' but it apparently aimed to target offenders, ex-offenders, drug users, young offenders, the physically disabled, the elderly and the sensory impaired. How could they think they were supporting the sight impaired when they were lumping us together with offenders, ex-offenders, young offenders and drug users? Sight impairment is a disability, not a criminal offence. (Or am I wrong?)

How could they think they were supporting the sight impaired when they were lumping us together with offenders and drug users?

I know I'm not alone in my frustration.

I know I'm not alone in my frustration. Times have changed and sight impaired people in Britain now have much higher aspirations than a century ago. Baby boomers are getting to an age where many of them are suffering sight problems and yet they are used to good service. Baby boom blindies will put organisations under the kind of pressure they haven't experienced to date. We baby boom blindies feel insulted at having to endure the cold and discomfort of draughty church hall meetings and we are not prepared to live out the rest of our lives as second-class citizens. We know we deserve better and we're beginning to demand it.

Chapter 37:

The blind leading the sighted

Perhaps the problem is that more often than not it's not sight impaired people who set the agenda. The thoughts and feelings of people with sight problems are often ignored because many organisations are run by well-intentioned sighted people. With the best will in the world, these sighted people cannot know what's best for people with sight impairment, nor can they be as motivated when it comes to campaigning for change. And very often they are frightened of saying the really hard things that might upset the sighted world, the people who give us our funding. Amongst themselves, they disagree about the best approach to take and waste time with infighting and political wrangling. Meanwhile, the people who have a problem with their eyesight can't campaign, precisely because of the lack of progress made.

In many ways I'm lucky because as well as being very confident I've also had a good education and a broad range of life experiences. However, I'm not typical, as one very shocking comment I overheard illustrated. One sighted executive charity worker turned to another and said 'He's very bright for a blind man, isn't he?' This is unforgivable! To hear someone so high up utter such a phrase makes my blood boil.

The sad fact is that there are many people in my world who haven't had my advantages. These people have no voice, no confidence and poor communication skills.

Many people haven't had my advantages.

Sometimes they are simply unable to put forward their own case in an effective way because their emotions overwhelm their attempts to argue rationally. For example, I once attended a meeting where the attendees were given the opportunity to lobby the European Transport Minister. One sight impaired gentleman spoke up but it soon emerged that he had neither the subject knowledge nor the eloquence to deal with the situation. When he realised he was losing the argument, he blurted out that he'd never in fact liked the minister and thought he was a 'fat bastard'. The minister and his entourage simply left the building and I for one don't blame him.

The deaf community always had such strong campaigners – campaigners like Jack (now Lord) Ashley. The sight impaired community, on the other hand, just had a few nice, middle-class, church-going ladies, with perfect eyesight, who could perhaps not put enough time or energy into campaigning. At least they started the ball rolling by setting up organisations such as the RNIB and Guide Dogs, but they haven't as yet made much progress.

To improve this situation sight impaired people need to be far more involved in leading an organised campaign, which is well supported by sighted people. We need to be working *alongside* sighted campaigners. To make this possible, we clearly need to improve education and training opportunities for people with any kind of sight impairment so that the sight impaired gradually develop the social, intellectual and managerial skills they need. The sight impaired also need to have leadership courses and skills development training so that fundraising can become more focused and professional. (And for that matter, why can't funds be provided so that professional fundraisers do the fundraising?) People with eyesight difficulties will then be in a much stronger position to present polite, yet effective campaigns, which will benefit enormously from any support the sighted community is also able to give. In this respect, I applaud the way in which Guide Dogs is being led by sight impaired people themselves and I would like to challenge sighted people within other charities to promote this model. All campaigns will be more effective if sight impaired people are at the helm. Who else has a better idea of what needs to be done?

We also desperately need the help of sighted people because too often sight impaired people don't act because of a lack of money, a lack of confidence and a lack of awareness of their own rights. As a result, I would urge sighted people within the RNIB and Guide Dogs to help bring forward class actions under DDA on behalf of all sight impaired people – the sighted are the ones with the resources and the influence. Failure to do so leaves sight impaired people disenfranchised.

Although I've always found politics to be mind-numbingly dull, I have become involved in this process of blindy-led campaigning. In recent years I've talked to parliamentary committees, individual Lords and MPs and I've even found myself marching outside parliament and speaking at a debate in Westminster Hall. Not bad for a blind lad from Jarrow! It certainly wasn't something I'd sought or expected, though. I'm now thinking of investing in my very own soapbox. And while I'm considering getting on it, I'd better mention right now that 'blindy' is a term only blindies are allowed to use. Don't try using it yourself. Believe me, it's not a good idea.

Chapter 38:

Soapbox

There's so much to say, it's difficult to know where to start. How about a few more statistics first of all? The RNIB tell us that 66% of sight impaired people are unemployed. 72% of those people live below the government's own poverty line. How can people in such circumstances access transport? No access to transport means no access to employment, less social engagement, which in turn leads to lives of segregation, isolation and loneliness.

As you might expect, there is a government allowance to help, at least a little. People who have a severe disability get an allowance known as the Disability Living Allowance (DLA). This has two components: the care component and the mobility component and the latter has two rates, one 'high' and one 'low'. The high rate is based on how far a person can walk unaided and blind and sight impaired people are currently only awarded the low rate. In other words, sight impairment is not usually regarded as something that impairs a person's ability to walk unaided. Does this make any sense at all? I would say that if an individual needs a dog, a long cane or a sighted guide in order to walk safely, he or she is not walking unaided. So why aren't blind or sight impaired people eligible for the higher rate? How can they be expected to get around and have a normal life on an allowance which is currently around £17 a week? According to the RNIB, 48% of sight impaired people admit they have difficulty going out alone because of potential hazards on the streets, as well as a lack of access to public transport.

I have enormous problems financing travel...

To give you an idea, here's a little information about my own transport costs. I now run my own business and I need to visit clients all over the region and beyond. Often I need to visit several clients in one day, just as many other businessmen do. I need to do this by taxi because I usually need to take along a laptop, projector, screen and briefcase – which certainly can't be carried in one hand, while holding a guide dog's lead with the other. This means I often have a weekly taxi bill of over £150, for work alone.

Shopping and entertainment are also difficult since many shopping centres, retail parks, entertainment complexes and DIY stores are out of town and accessible only by car.

Finally, I have enormous problems financing travel to family and friends. My parents, who are both well into their 70s, live on an estate with no bus service whatsoever, since it was recently discontinued. This means visiting them involves taxi rides totalling over £18... so one visit to see Mum and Dad more than blows my entire week's transport budget.

And how am I supposed to get to the folk club I've attended on and off for over 30 years? It doesn't begin until 8pm and the last bus home is at 8.30pm, but it hardly seems worth going for half an hour. On the other hand, the taxi ride there and back costs over £40. This means I only end up going when there's someone performing that Denise wants to see or when I'm feeling especially wealthy.

How am I supposed to get to the folk club?

The thing I find most frustrating is not being able to make a journey on the spur of the moment. In the old days I could take off somewhere purely on a whim and just hop on a bus or train and just go. Now I can't read timetables or guide books and signage is very often difficult, so all journeys – even the shortest – need careful planning. Travelling alone is also becoming increasingly difficult because so many places are inaccessible to me without someone to take me there. Denise or various friends and relatives often offer me lifts. This is wonderful but of course it means that journeys have to be made at other people's convenience, not mine, which I find extremely frustrating. And when I put pressure on people to go to places they have no interest in I end up feeling I'm a burden.

So, you see, the £17 weekly allowance I receive is in no way adequate compensation for the difficulties and expenses I incur. And when either the people to help me or the additional money aren't available I simply lose the right to free and easy movement.

Even people who are close to me often don't understand this point. I once got into a row with a very dear friend when I was banging on about this issue of mobility allowance. I was trying to explain how upset I feel at not being able to drive. I know why it's not possible, but it still hurts me deeply because it seems so incredibly unfair. Why should I have to walk Abbot through areas that have a bad reputation, feeling frightened and vulnerable, while other people drive through them safely, in locked cars? My friend argued that there are plenty of other people in our society who can't afford a car.

The point, though, is mainly to do with aspiration and freedom, both of which are linked to finance, of course. In terms of aspiration, even people who can't afford a car at the moment can aspire to owning one in the future. (While people's finances change over time, sight impairment is with a person for life.) And in terms of freedom, not owning a car is so limiting. This is because our society is increasingly geared towards drivers – so much so that driving is almost considered a right, from which sight impaired people are excluded.

We can narrow the gap between sight impaired and sighted people by compensating people better financially.

Although this is not a situation we can equalise, we can certainly narrow the gap between sight impaired and sighted people by compensating people better financially when they cannot drive because of sight impairment. People who can't see too well at least deserve the right to use public transport, or taxis in cases where no adequate public transport is available. And public transport could be made far more user-friendly, with better lighting, clearer markings and easier access.

STOP PRESS!
I've just had a phone call to tell me that legislation has just gone through parliament. This will mean that all severely sight impaired people will receive the higher rate of the mobility allowance from April 2011. About time!

Chapter 39:

Disabled, disadvantaged, abused (DDA)

Even if sight impaired people manage to get to a place, it's not always easy to get a reasonable level of service. The DDA (Disability Discrimination Act) makes it illegal to refuse service or offer a lesser service to sight impaired people just because it takes them longer to make their purchases. (This means service providers can't charge a sight impaired person more in order to meet the costs of providing any services – so, for example, an airline can't charge extra for a guide dog.) Similarly, it's illegal for a service provider to run a service in a way that makes it impossible or unreasonably difficult for a sight impaired person to use – unless a particular aspect of a service is considered to be fundamental to the business (e.g. dim lighting in the case of a nightclub.). This means that museums have to provide equipment which gives sight impaired people access to exhibits, such as an audio guide, and it also means that all physical barriers to access have to be removed. For the same reasons of access, a restaurant which generally does not admit animals cannot refuse access to a guide dog owner and his or her dog.

This reminds me of an incident in a pub one evening. The barman told me there were two women on the premises who were afraid of dogs. He told me he knew he couldn't ask me to leave but wondered if I might move on to another pub as one of these ladies was starting to panic. I finished my drink and left. I don't want to be in a place under those circumstances... But it should have been the ladies who left, not me. All my friends now boycott this pub and, believe me, they can drink! So who's the loser? Actually, if I'd really felt I'd been wrongly excluded from 'the provision of goods and service' I could have taken action through the courts. I may then have been awarded damages for any financial loss suffered or for injury to my feelings. Interestingly, no limit is placed on the amount of damages that can be paid for hurt feelings.

No limit is placed on the amount of damages that can be paid for hurt feelings.

I heard about one local guide dog owner who was going to meet his girlfriend's family for the first time. They had arranged to meet inside a local restaurant. By the time he and his dog arrived the rest of the party were already inside but the manager refused to let him in with his dog. Naturally, my friend was angry but he was reluctant to cause a scene because he wanted to make a good impression with his potential in-laws. He explained to the manager that his girlfriend and her family were already inside and asked if he would let them know. The manager went on to ask him what they looked like. He was so hurt he took the matter to court. He was awarded £13,000 in damages for hurt feelings.

In case you feel like hurting my feelings I've devised a little scale. Let's make 'Four eyes!' a bargain insult and just charge £100. And if you say 'You blind bastard!' I'll expect the full £13,000. Everything in between is negotiable.

Other people have other approaches... One guide dog owner was refused entry to a well-known burger bar.

He returned home and called their head office to complain. He was duly sent 12 free meal vouchers so he rounded up 11 of his guide dog owner friends and they all climbed on board a minibus and took themselves and their dogs back to the original burger bar. Personally, I'd have gone to court in search of a settlement.

In any case, if any standards are going to be enforced, the government needs to consider precisely *how*. Dedicated disabled seating on buses tends to get occupied by able-bodied passengers who will then not give up those seats when disabled people get on board. Bus drivers are reluctant to get involved so who is going to stand up for disabled passengers? Anyone with a complaint – on a bus or even in the workplace – should have access to a tribunal.

Now you may be thinking at this point 'Well, why should they bloody well get preferential treatment? What useful contribution can they possibly make to society?' Actually, I'm mainly asking for *equal* treatment and only 'preferential' in the sense that adjustments will sometimes need to be made just so that we blindies can have equal access. And as for the business of whether or not we're making a useful contribution to society, perhaps I'd better tell you the outcome to that conversation I had at the Job Centre about coat hangers...

Eventually, after some thought I decided I'd enrol for a BEd course so I could become a primary school teacher. Things were going swimmingly for most of the three year course, but then towards the end I started repeatedly having blackouts. (There was much dispute at the time between my consultants over whether it was my heart or my eyes that were causing the problem.)

Anyway, I was eventually told I might as well give up the teaching idea because I'd never be allowed into a classroom on my own.

As luck would have it, the DSS were having a massive recruitment drive at the time, so I signed up. I did almost four years with them, working on renewable one-year contracts dealing first with child support, then overseas benefits and eventually fraud investigation. It was only when I asked for five weeks of unpaid leave towards the end of the fourth contract (so I could do the guide dog training) that I had to stop doing this job... and become unemployed for the next 18 months.

> **Even with eye conditions, people can make a contribution. There's lots they can do.**

So, you see, even with eye conditions, people can make a contribution. There are lots of things they can do, even if they can't see too well any more. James Galway, one of the most famous musicians worldwide, has nystagmus. Nevertheless he's made a fantastic career out of playing the flute. Surely, other people with eyesight problems could make more of a contribution too, if only they were given more equal access to transport, facilities and job opportunities... We're sight impaired, you know, not daft.

Chapter 40:

Art lover

Over the last few years I've managed to create a job for myself in the field of sight impairment. My core work is in the area of access audit, which means checking buildings and public spaces to make them safe for sight impaired people to use. Most buildings and public spaces contain hazards that you may not have noticed. Let me take you on an imaginary audit round a local art gallery. All the details and incidents described here have actually been included in audit reports, but not all in the same one. I've just put them all together for the sake of illustration.

By the way, in case you're wondering why a man with a sight impairment might want to go to an art gallery, please let me remind you it's only my eyesight that's failing... I haven't had a cultural bypass. In fact, I love art, good design, literature and music and I don't think sight impairment should be a bar to any of the arts as long as a little sight remains. All the arts receive funding from government, the lottery and other bodies that represent everyone in society. If we're all paying, shouldn't we all have equal access?

Shouldn't we all have equal access?

As I approach the gallery's main entrance I encounter a set of 'A' boards blocking the path, set up right in front of the main entrance. On the path I see some broken glass, which is obviously a hazard to Abbot (as well as to all kinds of other people).

Entering the building, I point this out to a member of staff and mention that the glass needs to be cleared away. (An hour and a half later it's still there.)

In the foyer itself, which is used as a shop, there are too many display stands in too small a space, so I have trouble negotiating a path through. The aisles are so narrow that Abbot has to walk behind me. With him walking in the rear, I am now guiding him... Somehow, I don't think that was the idea.

To reach the main body of the gallery I have to climb a short flight of wooden stairs. The nosing on these stairs is brown and doesn't stand out against the wood. (It's all very well having nosing that's slip- and trip-resistant but why not make it helpful for people with sight problems, at no extra cost? Some colour contrast, please, Mr Curator.) I notice there is overhead lighting above the stairs but no one has bothered to turn it on.

Having moved from lino in the foyer to wood on the stairs, I then have to deal with a third change of surface at the top of the stairs, where I suddenly encounter marble. What many sight impaired people do is take note of the surface as they enter a room by rubbing a foot discretely on the floor as they pass through a door. When a surface changes within a room, where the sight impaired person is not expecting a change, this is a trip hazard. This type of hazard has caught me out on many occasions and made me fall over.

This type of hazard has caught me out many times and made me fall over.

On this small landing, at the top of the first flight of stairs, I realise that the master staircase is still to come. Rather unexpectedly, it's located to my right and there's no sign to help me find my way. This main staircase leads to other gallery spaces and the stairs have no nosing at all. For someone with poor depth perception, judging the gap between stairs without nosing is difficult, especially since – as before – these stairs are poorly lit.

The top of the stairs brings me into a lobby which doubles up as a gallery space. Here, as elsewhere in the building, I find the signage poor so it's difficult to work out where to go. Each of the exhibits has a small placard bearing relevant information but all the cards are written in Times New Roman 12 point. This particular font – a very common one – is difficult for sight impaired people to read as it has lots of tails and curls. 12 point is also far too small for many people with any kind of sight impairment. To make matters worse, the floor in this area is grey. About a foot above the floor there is a thin grey trip wire about six inches from the wall to stop people getting too close to the exhibits. (Grey floor plus grey wire means an accident waiting to happen.) I trip over the wire as I'm trying to get close enough to read the sign...

In the main galleries the same unhelpful colour scheme, trip wire and poor signage is repeated on a much grander scale. (Walls are painted either grey, dark red or bottle green, meaning there is constantly a lack of colour contrast with the wires.) The walls in these galleries are about 12 feet high and are covered floor to ceiling in pictures. The only ones that are accessible to sight impaired people are those at eye level. How difficult would it be to design walls which revolve like a turntable?

A whole wall could be rotated and pictures beyond eye level could then be brought into view. (Incidentally, one gallery used to have a range of tactile exhibits for sight impaired people but they were sold off and the money given to blind charities. I would have much preferred to see the exhibits remain within the gallery as a resource for the sight impaired community.)

Following the natural route through the gallery, I eventually come to another staircase that leads me back to the ground floor. This staircase is even darker than the others and, again, there is no nosing. (This issue was highlighted in an access audit six years before this visit, but still nothing has been done. Does this not already say something about the esteem the gallery has for sight impaired people? If there is a problem that can be easily rectified at little cost and yet it remains unresolved for over six years we can only assume that sight impaired people are not a priority.)

After making my way down the last staircase I find myself in a corridor that runs through the whole ground floor of the building. Some thoughtful person has decided that it would be a good idea to place plinths in the middle of the narrow corridor and stand exhibits on them. I accidentally walk into a few and panic as the exhibits wobble dangerously close to the edge.

The corridor eventually brings me to the gallery's coffee shop where I am confronted with a whole new set of problems. On entering, the first thing I notice is that there are too many tables and chairs in too small a space. This means there are no access routes between tables. (Once again Abbot has to follow behind and once again, I have to guide him.)

When I finally find my way to the counter I see that the menu is written by hand on a blackboard at ceiling height, about 15 feet up. As in the burger bar I mentioned in an earlier chapter, I stand there with Abbot in harness and ask what's on the menu only to be told 'It's up there.'

After I eventually manage to order something and sit down, I hear two of the staff loudly discussing my sight impairment. (Is this good customer care or what?!) After a while one of them approaches my table and proceeds to stroke Abbot without asking my permission first. Even worse, she then brings her face within inches of my own to see if I can see her. Perhaps, by now, you can understand how offensive this is.

The whole place seems to be designed to make people with a sight impairment struggle. Needless to say, my access audit report is not going to be positive.

If you have responsibility for a building or public space, please think about access, lighting, signage, stairs and above all staff training. If you're unsure whether your premises meet the standards required by DDA, consult an access auditor. Make sure that your auditor doesn't just look at the needs of the physically disabled and that he or she also checks for the needs of the sensory impaired. Far too many auditors are not good at this. If you need one, I know this bloke with a guide dog...

If you're unsure whether your premises meet the standards required, consult an auditor.

Chapter 41:

Dark days

Back in my ordinary life, I'm having a good day. One of the best, in fact. The sun is shining and Denise and I are out shopping. For a long time before Abbot arrived I'd stopped going out like this, so this is a real treat. I've really missed days like this, little bits of normality, frittering time, wandering aimlessly and chatting about nothing in particular – days when we can simply daydream a little, wander round the shops and maybe stop for a coffee. I always feel that Denise and I have our best conversations while we're out for coffee as there are none of the interruptions of home, no phone calls, no email, no tasks awaiting my attention. Days like this are all too rare and I value them beyond measure. Today is one of those days.

Abbot is in top form, his tail is up and he's working well, weaving his way through the crowds, the thing he loves most. He's getting lots of admiring glances. As for me, I'm on a little high, cracking jokes and prattling on about any old rubbish... But who can tell what's about to hit, right out of a clear blue sky?

We leave the shops with armfuls of shopping so we decide to get a taxi home. I call the taxi company and explain to the girl on the desk that I have my guide dog with me. (As I've explained, I have the legal right to take my dog in a cab but I always let the taxi company know in advance because I think it's the courteous thing to do.) The girl assures me it's fine, I hang up and go outside to wait with Denise.

"No fucking dog is getting in my taxi."

When the taxi arrives the driver springs out of the car:

"That's a fucking dog!" he screams.

"It's a guide dog", I reply.

"I don't give a shit. No fucking dog is getting in my fucking taxi."

Some drivers have allergies and the law requires them to carry an exemption certificate. I ask if he has one. His response is 'Fuck off'. I remind him that unless he has a certificate, he's breaking the law. That seems to get his attention and he agrees to take us, even though I'm apparently still a fucking idiot. I decline and he speeds off, still hurling abuse out of the window as he pulls away.

While all this has been going on a small crowd has gathered. People are pointing and craning their necks to see what all the fuss is about. Denise and I both feel we're at the centre of a freak show. But there is more to come, from a source I'd never have expected.

My guide dog owner's manual (I kid you not) gives clear guidelines on how to proceed in such situations. (It's right near the back, just before the bit on how to change the oil. OK, OK. I am joking now.) The manual tells us to simply remove ourselves from the situation and report to Guide Dogs. So that's exactly what I do, as soon as I get home, using another taxi company. To my astonishment, Guide Dogs replies that as long as I got home safely they don't really want to take up the issue with the offending taxi firm.

This one incident sets us back months. Denise, unlike her husband, is a very shy and private person. She says she feels less conspicuous shopping on her own. She doesn't want to run the risk of another incident. I, on the other hand, feel I'm missing out on quality time with her. I begin to question my decision to get Abbot. All my worst fears about being abused by the public have come true. This has to be my lowest point in my time with Abbot.

I flatly refuse to leave the house. Friends and family all try hard to coax me to.

For almost a month I flatly refuse to leave the house. Friends and family all try hard to coax me out of my self-imposed confinement but I refuse to be persuaded. I just feel too embarrassed. God knows, I have a huge ego but this was never the type of attention I craved. We're back in nightmare country and my running shoes have come out of storage.

The good thing is that I'm so in love with Abbot I can't cope with the idea of handing him back to Guide Dogs. So I eventually force myself back out onto the streets with my boy, even though my confidence is badly shaken. I spend the first few outings waiting for someone to object to Abbot's presence or otherwise abuse me. This is not the confident and empowered me that was here just a few short weeks ago. What used to be such good fun now seems like my worst nightmare and it takes several months to get my confidence back. A life tied to the house suddenly seems more attractive than running the risk of taking abuse out there on the street.

The government is doing something right... Long may it continue.

If someone as confident as me, with a big mouth, a big ego and an even bigger head can feel so low, what hope is there for someone of a more nervous disposition? Too many sight impaired people are becoming housebound for exactly this reason. This cannot be allowed to continue. Realising this, I summon up all my courage and contact my local council. The offending taxi driver is suspended for a month and sent for low vision awareness training. So the government is doing something right, I admit. Long may it continue.

Chapter 42:

Walk the dog

Let me tell you a bit more about puppy walking. My friend Ethne, who comes with me to give talks for Guide Dogs, has now walked over a dozen dogs. Ethne and all puppy walkers have my greatest respect, as do all Guide Dogs' 10,000 volunteers, who include puppy walkers, brood-stock holders, dog boarders and local fundraisers.

The work puppy walkers do is particularly important to people like me and it's all done on a voluntary basis. They give a great deal of time, love and patience, not to mention money, to the rearing of the 1,000 or so puppies which Guide Dogs breed each year. It's their job to acclimatise the pups to everyday situations such as shops, pubs, restaurants, buses and trains, etc. For a whole year, the puppy is their third arm: wherever they go, pup goes too. Then after 12 months of love, tears and downright hard work they have to give it up. This is a real commitment and it's exactly why I hold puppy walkers in the highest regard.

Abbot's puppy walkers, Jan and Mick, were wonderfully dedicated people whose love and commitment shine out through Abbot. I hope they're as proud of him as I am, as all the credit belongs to them.

Abbot has many fine qualities, which I attribute directly to Jan and Mick... He's a very loving dog who adores a fuss, yet he never makes a nuisance of himself. His social behaviour is impeccable and I never need to worry, no matter what the situation. In church he sits under the pew and you wouldn't know he was there. I spend my life constantly in meetings and many times no one has known he was there until the meeting was over and I brought him out from under the table as we got ready to leave.

We did have one memorable incident, though. We were out for a meal and as usual Abbot was under the table, minding his own business. The waitress made her way between the tables with a tray of Yorkshire puddings, when suddenly she threw the tray up in the air and screamed. She fixed me with a look of contempt and as she raised her hand to slap me, Abbot popped out from under the table to see what was going on. It had been his cold black nose under her mini skirt that had caused all the commotion. Immediately, the waitress recoiled and started to laugh. That was a close one, I thought. Never one to miss an opportunity, Abbot deftly hoovered up the Yorkshire puddings.

Getting back to puppy walkers, who make sure this kind of thing rarely happens, they are recruited in all kinds of interesting ways. Once a man spotted me in a supermarket and after taking one look at Abbot, he burst into tears. He explained that he'd just lost a dog that looked just like Abbot. He died after a long illness and seeing Abbot had brought it all back. We'd caught him at a low ebb. We talked at length about the pain and pleasure of dog ownership. After a while I asked him if he'd ever thought about puppy walking. He thought that giving a puppy up would be just too painful. Not one to be put off easily, I asked him if he'd ever seen a guide dog at work. He hadn't, so I told him to follow me. I worked Abbot all round the supermarket for about twenty minutes and we eventually ended up where we started.

When we stopped I noticed the man was in tears again. He said it was fantastic but he still didn't know about having to give them up. I explained that giving a dog up to work for a blind person has to be a better feeling than losing a dog to ill health. He told me I'd given him some food for thought and we parted company. A few weeks later I heard through Guide Dogs that he was already walking his first puppy.

He told me I'd given him some food for thought and we parted company.

Getting back to Ethne, I have such enormous trust in her that she's now the only person I would trust to look after Abbot. Ethne's house is where Abbot goes for his holidays. Whenever I have to go away and can't take Abbot with me, he goes to his Auntie Ethne's house. She knows the rules and I know that when I get back his work will be bang up to the mark.

One more comment, in case you're thinking those sad-looking guide dogs need more holidays: Abbot really does live to work – as do other guide dogs, no doubt. If I show him his flexi-lead, which means that he gets to go out and play in a field with a friend of mine, and I also show him his harness, Abbot will always opt for the harness and his tail will go into demented helicopter mode. So those puppy walkers are not preparing the dogs for a life of drudgery – the dogs really do seem to enjoy being trained up and given a useful working life. I suppose, like Abbot, I would also prefer to do something useful than laze around catching up on sleep.

Chapter 43:

Mixed messages

Every evening as we arrive home, Abbot gives the gatepost a little sniff. Someone once told me he was just collecting his pee-mail – or p-mail. I liked this idea a lot and I've been giving the matter some thought. Abbot's p-mail comes in a form that's easily accessible to him. Oh, that all my messages were that easy to access. Abbot doesn't need anyone to read his messages for him and thank God for that! Nor does he require any fancy software to decipher them. If only it was that simple for sight impaired people.

We live in a digital age of email, text messaging and Internet use, none of which were originally designed to accommodate the needs of sight impaired people. It's all too easy to begin to feel excluded when so many people in society have such easy access to these forms of communication and paranoia can set in. Please don't misunderstand me here. I don't begrudge anyone access to such methods of communication. I would just like to see it made easier for sight impaired people to access these services at the same cost. All too often the equipment a sight impaired person might need (such as speech software or an accessible mobile phone) is prohibitively expensive. I would also like to see society have a better understanding of the issues facing sight impaired people around emailing, texting and the use of websites.

Equipment is often prohibitively expensive.

Let's deal with texting first. Normal size text is almost impossible for sight impaired people to deal with. Phones with talking text are often two or three times the price of a standard phone. Nowadays texting is often used as the only way of communicating with an organisation or individual, and this is a discriminatory practice. Radio and TV stations have competitions where the only way to take part is by text. And sometimes individuals wrongly assume we all have equal access to text messages. I once received a very angry phone call from someone at a local charity asking why I hadn't responded to several text messages he'd sent. The answer was quite simple: I couldn't see well enough to read them. I reminded him that I'm registered severely sight impaired and a guide dog owner too. He already knew this but he simply wasn't thinking. (I've discovered that some people are like computers: they need to have information punched into them.)

Email is not quite so difficult to deal with but there are still many sight impaired people who need extra software in order to deal with it. Again, this is often prohibitively expensive. I use speech software which is probably the most commonly used type amongst the blind community and it cost me over £1,300 in 2006 – a time when it was possible to buy a computer for £200.

Then there's the thorny issue of websites, which many sight impaired people can only use with the help of speech software. Much of this software can't cope with sites which contain lots of images and graphics. This means that many sight impaired people who rely on the little of their eyesight which remains find such sites very difficult to use... they're just too fussy and cluttered to be easily readable.

Many websites have made attempts to try and cope with these issues by introducing text-only sites. Although you may think this is helpful and they may fulfil some access needs they fail on grounds of equality – and if it's an organisation with an equality policy it may well be in breach of its own policy. To simply leave out images and graphics that are available on the main site is not an equality option. It can leave a sight impaired person wondering what they might be missing, so again it can lead to feelings of isolation and paranoia.

As for p-mail, I'm sure it works just fine for Abbot and his mates, but somehow I just don't fancy it. You could say I'm a bit sniffy about it.

Although you may think text-only sites are helpful, they fail on grounds of equality.

Chapter 44:

We'll just write

Snail mail from official bodies is a particular problem. Neither central nor local government seem to use the sight impairment register to really help sight impaired people. Nevertheless, they're doing a wonderful job of using it to fuel frustration.

For example, I sometimes get letters and forms from the Inland Revenue. Although I've now officially been on the sight impairment register for nine years, this government organisation still fails to correspond with me in my preferred format (large print). As a result, I have to ask Denise to read the paperwork to me.

When I set up my own business a couple of years ago, those nice people at the Inland Revenue also sent me a Starter Pack... in normal print. (The print was so small that even Denise had difficulty reading it.) Being the shy and retiring type, I rang them up and asked if I could have the pack in large print. The man who answered the phone said he wasn't sure if this was possible. Why did they ask for my preferred format, I wondered, if they had no intention of providing it?

Three days later I got a phone call. It might just be possible to get me a large print copy, the man said... a copy that is my legal right to receive in accordance with DDA. He then went on to ask why a blind man wanted to start a business. How bloody rude!

Two years on I'm still waiting for my large print guide from the Inland Revenue. Would they wait two years for me to pay my tax?

I've also had a few frustrating interactions with the Criminal Records Bureau (the CRB) over the last four years. They refuse to provide forms in accessible formats, but in doing so I feel they're in breach of DDA. After all, I can't think of any other form that is as personal and as private as a CRB form.

As well as rude, insulting and extremely frustrating, these communications from government agencies are also rather odd. The DDA clearly states that public bodies must make 'reasonable adjustment' for people's disability but surely providing information in my preferred format would come under this term? (Who wrote the DDA, by the way? Yes, that's right: the government.)

At least the government are not alone here. There are many service providers who don't provide sight impaired people with written materials in other formats either at all or within a reasonable timeframe. A general rule for written materials should be that all forms or standard letters should be held in stock so that sight impaired people receive their copies within the same timescale as sighted people. If it's a bespoke item, such as a letter which is personal and specific to that sight impaired person, then a short delay may be acceptable. In addition, companies which send literature out to clients should already have a supplier in place who can provide documents in other formats. It's no good waiting till you get a request and then scratching around trying to find a supplier as this will cause unnecessary and unacceptable delay.

And what kind of written materials are appropriate? The guidelines are really quite simple...

It's helpful to use a sans serif font (such as Arial or Verdana), a point size which is at least 14 point (or preferably 16 point), easy-to-read headings, plenty of contrast (e.g. dark lettering on a very light background), clear captions on photographs and a straightforward but attractive layout. Not too difficult, is it? I believe those who fail to grasp this will be left behind commercially. After all, companies who make their literature inaccessible are missing out on up to 40% of the UK population. If this surprises you, consider that according to the RNIB there are three million people in the UK with sight loss or dyslexia, who are unable to read 96% of regular literature. The RNIB also tell us that for every person registered as sight impaired there are another two who simply refuse to do so. (They estimate that as many as 38% of the British population have a significant sight problem.) So it's a hidden epidemic. The BBC tells us that one in every three drivers has such poor sight they would not currently pass a driving test. Here, we're talking about people with glasses or contact lenses, people who are too vain to wear either and people who have difficulty reading a newspaper or watching TV. These are people who can't read sell-by dates or fill in a lottery ticket.

Consider all this in the light of the fact that (according to the Disability Rights Commission) organisations in the UK spend £20 billion a year communicating with their customer base. We need to think of the phrase 'clear print' as if it were a British Kitemark. Unless we do, how can we be sure that any potential customers will have equal equipment access to products and services? And how can we ensure that companies will have equal rights to profitability?

Chapter 45:

Onward!

The RNIB is campaigning for bigger, clearer print to be used in all printed materials. It's also campaigning for what it calls 'inclusive design' so that machines such as dishwashers and washing machines are usable by sight impaired people. This will include items such as computers, mobile phones and televisions so that they are all made more accessible to blind and sight impaired people. Olympus have already followed their guidelines so as to produce easy-to-use recording equipment.

Under the DDA, other changes are also being made. Since the end of 2009, on all buses in London recorded information about destinations and stops has been relayed to all passengers. Nationally, all new trains built after 1998 are meant by law to have audio-visual information in their carriages and all trains will have to have these systems in place no later than 2020.

There are problems which still need to be solved, though. For example, what will be done in cases where audio-visual systems in public transport have not been turned on, or are broken? There is as yet no statutory enforcement system in place. And what is being done for pedestrians? Urban planners currently favour a system known as 'naked streets', where kerbs are taken away and the distinction between street and road disappears. According to Guide Dogs, this is the most serious threat to the mobility of sight impaired people. After all, kerbs are the single most useful navigational tool for sight impaired people.

Employers' ignorance about government-funded Access To Work benefits is also a major stumbling block to progress, according to the RNIB. Most employers are unaware that government funding is available to pay for additional help, adaptations and software designed to help a sight impaired person in the workplace.

To make matters worse, the RNIB says that employers make false assumptions about what sight impaired people are capable of. They say that a lot of employers take the stereotypical view that if you have a sight impairment you can only be a telephonist or tune pianos. The RNIB say employers need to turn that opinion on its head and instead think of a job which a sight impaired person *can't* do.

Employment issues really do need to be addressed. After all, as we've already mentioned, too many sight impaired people of working age are unemployed — 66%, was the RNIB statistic, if you remember — and 67% of sight impaired people have no formal qualifications. Fazilet Hazi, RNIB Director of Policy and Advocacy says:

"[It] isn't just about changing the law. I think we should use the law and challenge it more. We also need to change the way people think."

Sue Sharpe, Head of Public Policy and Campaigns at Guide Dogs agrees:

"It's one thing having the legislation, it's another thing delivering it."

Again and again, I've experienced lack of information and accessibility on a very personal level. I've repeatedly felt myself being knocked down by either people or systems.

When I became unemployed, I did eventually muster the courage to tackle something else and I did find information...

Nevertheless, when I became unemployed after getting Abbot, I did eventually muster up the courage to tackle something else and in the end I did manage to find the relevant information. About a year later, with the help of a bank loan and Denise's support (who's always had a steady job), I enrolled in a distance learning MA in Access Audit with Leeds University. That's how I came to be able to set up the consultancy I now run.

Lack of access to information which makes this kind of life change difficult is a major problem for the sight impaired. (This includes lack of access to newspapers, books and the Internet, as well as instruction manuals for household appliances.) The information deficit which results stands in the way of equality of service, access to education and the performance of daily tasks, which sighted people take for granted.

Alongside the psychological trauma of sight impairment, this lack of access is another stress factor. Yes, there certainly are things people can do, even when their sight is failing, but how are they going to work out what they are when it's so difficult for them to access basic information and simply get from A to B?

Someone, somewhere really does need to think through the logistics of making DDA a reality for the sight impaired so we can work alongside the sighted community in a more collaborative and tolerant world.

Chapter 46:

Bad reception

It's now four years since I was registered severely sight impaired and my sight has deteriorated even more since then. Am I coping? Well, it makes me think of two things... First, there's music, as there always has been. Then there are memories of my childhood and adulthood, while I was slowly losing more and more of my eyesight.

Let's deal with the music first. I didn't think I had a song in my CD collection that dealt with how I've been feeling lately. Then I returned to my old friend Allan Taylor and his song 'Misty On The Water'. Allan sang:

You were misty on the water. You were foggy on the dawn. When I tried to follow after, I looked and found you gone. I looked and found you gone. Where could you be? When it's misty on the water, it's hard to see.

[Words and music by Allan Taylor. Used with kind permission.]

These lyrics sum up my sight these days. Sometimes the mist clears and I get a fleeting glimpse of clarity and just as I begin to celebrate, the mist rolls back and I'm left exiled.

As for the memories, I've been remembering camping holidays. I loved those camping trips we made when I was a child. We had a little black and white TV that worked off the car battery. We spent many an evening standing on deckchairs and climbing on camping tables, waving the aerial aloft, trying to get a better picture. There'd be shouts of delight when the screen cleared and a good picture was visible, then cries of woe when the person holding the aerial moved and the picture was lost and the screen filled with static again. That was 30 years ago or more, but my sight now reminds me of those days. I can spend all day in search of clear reception and then as fast as it comes, it's gone again.

I also remember a dream from those childhood days. It was a recurring dream that persisted throughout my childhood. In the dream I was always falling through the air past an enormous billboard. As I fell I was trying to read the endless lines of text on the board – but I was falling so fast that I was unable to decipher any of the messages. The falling in itself was not frightening... I was just so frustrated at not being able to read the message. I was falling so fast, the words were passing by my eyes too quickly for me to read them. I would wake up with the odd random word fixed in my mind but there were not enough words to make any sense of the message. This would leave me feeling deeply frustrated and confused.

Another memory comes to mind from more recent years. It reminds me more than ever what a difference Abbot has made to me. Not only has he extended my field of vision, he's also given me more confidence than I could ever have found without him. About six months before he arrived on the scene I was with the DSS (as I said), working as a fraud investigator. One day I had to inform a client that since he'd failed to sign on that week, he wouldn't get paid. He'd actually been found 'drunk and disorderly' the day before he was due to sign on and had spent the night in a police cell. When he was released the next day he'd already missed his signing appointment and unfortunately he didn't bother to contact us. This meant we couldn't legally give him his benefit cheque because technically he hadn't been available for work that day.

Some of the language he used when he came to see me was too much even for me. I'd include it here to give you an idea but I wouldn't even know how to spell it. The main point is that he issued many threats against me that day – but this was really par for the course in that job, so I didn't worry too much. Instead, I did my best to laugh it off and put it all out of my mind. It was certainly not the first time I'd been threatened like this.

The next morning I got off the bus as usual and was making my way through the office car park when I was suddenly hit on the side of the head. My client and several of his friends had approached from either side, beyond the scope of my peripheral vision. It was a dark winter's morning and these were far from ideal conditions for someone with nystagmus.

By the time I'd focused on my attackers it was far too late to run and I knew I was going to take a beating. For the next five minutes they used me as a human football and kicked me around the staff car park. They were eventually disturbed by the arrival of several of my colleagues. The incident concluded with me sitting in A&E with an arm broken in two places and my confidence in tatters. They plastered my arm and it healed in a few short weeks but my confidence would remain in pieces until Abbot's arrival almost 18 months later. I did manage to keep on going into work for another six months, but going out alone purely for pleasure simply didn't feature any longer. Friends would call and invite me to the pub or to a concert but I would make some lame excuse and stay at home.

A lot of people around me attributed my nervousness to a fear of being assaulted, but it wasn't that at all. It's true that I was afraid – but I was afraid of not being able to *see* approaching danger, not of the danger itself. I suppose it's the same kind of thing as sighted people being afraid of walking around in the dark.

I suppose it's the same as sighted people being afraid of walking around in the dark.

Once I did reluctantly agree to go out – to Newcastle city centre with a few of my workmates. We were walking through the big market area at closing time. There was a lot of shouting going on and a lot of bad language. Someone yelled, 'Dave!' It wasn't directed at me but as it came from outside my visual field it left me with a feeling of panic and dread.

While I can't pretend any of this isn't upsetting, I'm very aware that Denise, Abbot and everybody that loves me are watching out for me. I'm very moved by all their care. (I told you it was getting like *The Waltons*.)

If a person like me needs this kind of support (someone who is usually very confident and outgoing), whatever can it be like for a person who doesn't have any natural confidence in the first place? Does their sight loss mean they're condemned to a life of confinement in their own homes?

Chapter 47:

Speaking for myself

We're getting near the end now and I'm sure there must be some issue or other over which we disagree. You wouldn't be the first to tell me what a stubborn pain in the arse I can be. Don't worry... this is what I expected and you can't help being wrong. I want this book to be challenging. I want to encourage a debate on issues relating to sight impairment. Above all, I want to get the sighted community to walk a mile in the shoes of the sight impaired. If I can just change the mind of one sighted person, I'll consider this book a success.

I know there are people I may have been too harsh about. I've found it difficult to portray the issues without seeming overcritical and only you can decide if I've been successful. All I know is that if you think I've been too harsh, just be glad you didn't read an earlier draft. In earlier drafts, David Blunkett was kidnapped and held hostage until all blind people got top rate mobility allowance. I'd even contemplated the forced redundancy of the employees of a certain fast food company. Also, I was about to pass a law that would change the words of the nursery rhyme to 'three sight impaired mice'. Mind you, it wasn't all bad... I was also going to start a new charity called Eating Dogs for the Anorexic.

If you think I've been too harsh, just be glad you didn't read an earlier draft of this book.

Seriously though, some of my comments have been written in anger. I've tried to put this to one side so as to save face with you but in truth there are some subjects which are still too raw to comment on in a less passionate way. There are some subjects I'm so angry about I haven't dared include them here at all. And I certainly haven't learned to see the funny side of them.

The plain fact is that this is not a book written on behalf of anyone. I am not in the employ of any blind charity nor am I a spokesman for the sight impaired. I represent no one but myself and even then I'm prone to changing my own mind. I'm simply a blind man trying to come to terms with his own sight impairment and all the emotions that go with it – the good, the bad and the downright ugly.

You may not agree with my politics and – who knows? – you could be right. My interpretation of disability law may be a bit too militant for your tastes but I make no apology for it, nor will you be able to change my mind. This book is just my way of dealing with all these feelings and issues in a way that is true to myself. If it makes me look bad, that's probably because I am bad. What I have given you here are merely edited highlights. (I have been far too embarrassed to admit to some of my behaviour.)

Suffice to say, from that horrible day in 1987 onwards (when I lost my job in bakery management), I spent well over a decade in a blind fury – almost literally! I was in such a filthy temper about my sight loss that I didn't have a single thought about how my behaviour might impact on all those around me. After all, it was their fault!

There were years and years when my behaviour was simply unacceptable and the legacy of that period lives with me still. There are many people who were so hurt by my behaviour that they remain to this day unable to forgive me and move on. I cannot begin to describe how sad this makes me. These people are never far from my thoughts and I am deeply ashamed. My life is only redeemed by the love of Denise and Abbot, none of which I deserve but all of which I thank God for daily.

In the end I'm just a bad-tempered blindy from Jarrow, searching for something to make sense of this madness. I think I've started finding solutions, but it's a long road and who can say how it will end?

All I know is that with Abbot at my side, anything is possible. He came into my life when I was about to press the self-destruct button. Single-pawed, he has saved me from myself. God bless him and keep him safe. I owe him more than these feeble words can express.

However, because I don't want this to be a soppy, sugary, sentimental tale – but a true-life account which really conveys my feelings (which I know a lot of other blind people share) – I must add one thing here: I think it's time the sighted community stopped putting dogs before people. Yes, it's great that sighted people love guide dog puppies and guide dogs and that they make a huge fuss over Abbot and his doggy colleagues... but I wish they would learn to love and care for their owners as well. Often someone will bend down to make a fuss of Abbot saying 'Ah isn't he lovely?' to which I reply 'His owner's not bad either.'

It's time the sighted community stopped putting dogs before people.

By now, you should realise that this statement in no way dilutes my feelings about Abbot. But consider how I feel when I meet people who are greatly taken by Abbot and make passionate enquiries about his welfare without once ever asking about mine. Have you any idea how demeaning that can be? Can you imagine what that can do to the self-esteem of a guide dog owner? Of course it's good that so many people show such love for our dogs but sight impaired people need to be placed before their dogs in the concerns of everyone, always.

Guide Dogs for the Blind accepts this viewpoint. Despite its name, it's not a dog charity – it exists to serve the needs of sight impaired people and despite its cuddly image it is a campaigning body with a mandate to promote the independence of sight impaired people.

This is what must be kept at the forefront of the agenda and any volunteers who are only there because they love puppies are really in the wrong place. They should either move to another charity or refocus their attention on the sight impaired people who need them. It's great to appreciate and enjoy the dogs, but focusing on the human beings and understanding their needs and interests is much more important at the end of the day... and all through it, in fact!

Focusing on humans is more important..

Chapter 48:

Facing my fear

Today is 14 December and it's exactly seven years to the day since Abbot and I qualified as a partnership. Four weeks ago, Sue came out from Guide Dogs to give us our annual aftercare visit. As usual she parked the car a few streets away and phoned, telling us which route she wanted us to take. After half an hour of trudging round the back streets of downtown Jarrow we arrived back home and Sue came in to discuss things.

She informed me that it was now time to think about Abbot's retirement. I am now on a waiting list to find a new dog and Abbot will be allowed to continue working until a new match is found, a process which can take anything up to 18 months. In my head, I know that Sue's decision is the right one but this is not an intellectual exercise, it's a matter of the heart and in my heart I am in great conflict and confusion. I love Abbot and I know he deserves a long and happy retirement. That's one thing... but then, more than anything, I'm feeling sorry for myself. For all of the last seven years it's been 'The Abbot and Dave Show'. Now that we're about to take our final bow I find myself totally unprepared for the event. I'm a musician and I know that bands break up, but it's going to be painful.

Throughout Abbot's career I have promised myself that when this moment came I would be prepared for it and that I would handle it with grace and composure. But I was wrong. I'm totally unprepared and I feel far from gracious or composed. I want to scream at the world at the sheer unfairness of it all. I'm looking for a fight with anyone who'd be foolish enough to take me on while I'm in this frame of mind. He's my boy, my pride and joy. He's been at the centre of my universe for all these years and I don't want anything to change, although I know it must change.

Sue and I have talked at great length and I fully understand all her reasoning. I know she's right. Abbot will not be going anywhere and will stay on to see out his days with Denise and me and I know he will be spoiled rotten with love, affection, walks on the beach and maybe just the odd treat, just as he deserves. But there are all these other emotions rolling around my head too.

Sometimes I'm overwhelmed with feelings of guilt, a guilt that says maybe if I'd done something different, Abbot and I may have had a few more years together… When I apply my powers of logic to this thought I know these feelings make no sense at all, but logic has no place here. This is a relationship which is stronger by far than many human relationships. We've all known the pain and sadness that happens at the end of a friendship or a love affair. Relationships break down and sadly people die. And those of us left behind have to come to terms with our feelings of loss.

I feel that I'm maybe letting Abbot down, that maybe I haven't been as good an owner as I should have been. Part of the reasoning behind the decision to retire Abbot at what is a slightly early stage is the fact that my sight has deteriorated so greatly. When we first qualified, seven years ago, I had so much more useful sight than I do now. Abbot grew used to the level of vision I had and for him to adapt to my new circumstances at this late stage in his career would simply be too much to ask of the old boy. So I am sure that a certain amount of what I am feeling is a none-too-small amount of self pity for the deterioration in my sight.

That day when Sue came to assess us I tried extremely hard to hide the recent deterioration in my eyesight for fear that she would come to exactly this decision. For this reason, I'd practised walking nearby streets and I'd even memorised certain obstacles... But Sue is a wily old bird and she knew exactly what I was up to. There was simply no fooling her: the game was up. Now I am a true blindy – I can no longer fool the experts into thinking I can perhaps see more than I am able to. Only yesterday I went to see my consultant and while I thought he was preoccupied with a phone call I memorised some of the eye chart he'd foolishly left on the table at my side. He put down the phone, grinned at me and changed the chart. The bastard.

My, oh my! This new development is a severe blow to the old ego. It feels like defeat but it's a defeat I can now come to terms with. Seven years ago I would not have been able to handle the news of Abbot's retirement and I owe all that to Abbot. Even now that he is about to retire he is still teaching me, leading me forward and looking after me. I love the old boy more than you'll ever know. Most of all, this feels like a bereavement – a bereavement where the other person is suffering a long illness, an illness that both people know will end badly, but which neither one can bring themselves to talk about.

My, oh my! This feels like a bereavement.

All I can say is that I know it's the right decision but it's bloody hard. However, of all the things Abbot has taught me, the biggest is that we face all our obstacles together and this is just another obstacle we'll face together. I'm sure we'll overcome it, just like all the others. We're brothers, forever. In the immortal words of Buzz Lightyear: 'To infinity and beyond!' Even in retirement Abbot will be ever at my side, teaching me, encouraging me, leading me forward.

> Even in retirement Abbot will be ever at my side, teaching me, encouraging me, leading me forward.

Chapter 49:

Why do I love him?

I love the way Abbot fills a room. His presence is a tangible thing. When he enters a room I can almost hear him shout 'TA DA!'

I love the way he leaps into our bedroom as it begins to get light. Every day is a brand new adventure to him and his enthusiasm is infectious. Even on a cold winter's morning at six o'clock Abbot bounds into the room at the sound of the alarm, ready for a new set of mischief and it makes me grin.

Days when my sight is worst and depression is tapping on my shoulder, Abbot will deposit a toy at my feet as if to say 'Stuff them, Dad.' Who could stay unhappy when my boy is grinning at them?

Abbot has an in-built sense of when my sight is particularly poor. He slows his pace down, he moves in close to my leg and I can feel the twist in his harness as he looks up to check if I'm OK. I can hear my gran whisper 'Good lad.'

I love walking him through a busy shopping area. These used to be the places I was most frightened of. Now I can almost hear him shouting 'Coming through!' The crowds part and he gives a little swagger. And I sometimes go out in the dark just because I can. I used to be scared of the dark like a child is scared of the bogeyman. Now Abbot has reclaimed the darkness.

I love 8 o'clock in the evening, which is 'treat time'. Abbot will go and sit by the cupboard and point with his nose: 'It's in there, Dad.'

I love watching him sleep too. Abbot's dream life seems very exciting. I don't know what goes on in his dreams but I've spent many happy hours just watching him.

> He's such a happy lad. In seven years I've never seen him in a grumpy mood.

He's such a happy lad. In seven years I've never seen him in a grumpy mood. He throws himself into everything with boundless enthusiasm. Most of all, I just love the fact that he's still a real dog. He loves to do the things all dogs do: tail-chasing, running and playing, getting into mischief... I just love it. He's far from being just a mobility tool. He's a free-thinking, sentient being who works for me out of choice, out of love – and it's a love that is mutual and deeply felt. No one has ever mistreated him in any way. Abbot was reared and trained by kindness and it's kindness that he responds to. He works for me because he cares deeply for me in the same way that I care for him. We're brothers – a true partnership built on mutual love and respect. Every time he puts on his harness and comes to work it's out of choice. He gives freely and I very gratefully accept. As my friend Ethne will tell you, we're the perfect match... we're both nutters.

Many dog owners will tell you they have the best dog in the world. They're bloody liars. I have.

> We're brothers — a true partnership.

Chapter 50:

The abbot's rule

As I mentioned before, I've always had an interest in Celtic Christianity and the monastic life. Traditionally, monastic communities live by a rule, which is laid down by the abbot. This rule is like a mission statement and it expresses their raison d'être.

In true monastic tradition Abbot has given us a rule to live by, which is as profound as any I've seen. We, his humble followers, should aspire to it, so here it is:

- Always greet those you love with warmth and enthusiasm. Don't be standoffish, dive straight in and nuzzle them. Roll onto your back and let them tickle your tummy. When someone new comes through the door, find them a present and stick it in their face.

- If those you love are going out on an adventure, make it quite obvious you'd like to go too. Don't wait to be asked. Shy bairns get nowt, as my dad says. Go and sit at the front door so they don't forget you.

- Savour pleasures such as fresh air, the wind in your face, a run on the beach and – with luck – a dip in the sea, even in December.

- Be obedient, especially if there's food on offer. It always works for my owner – you should see the size of him!

Always greet those you love with warmth.

- When someone has invaded your space, growl at them gently. Let them know where the boundaries are but don't hold a grudge.

- Take plenty of naps. You can't beat a good snooze and no one can overdo it. Find the best spot in the garden and stretch out in it. When you wake up, have a good stretch, then a scratch and maybe even a shake.

- Run, bounce around and play every day. Encourage all those around you to join in. Don't take 'no' for an answer. Gently take hold of each person's wrist and drag them into the game.

- Thrive on attention and let people make plenty of fuss of you. This has always worked well for me. Do your best to look cute.

- If you get told off or shouted at, don't sulk. Go straight back and make friends.

- Eat with great enthusiasm. When you've had enough stop, burp and have a nap.

- Be loyal, but never pretend to be something you're not.

- If what you want is buried, go digging for it. Don't stop until you find it.

- When someone's having a bad day, sit close, stay quiet and nuzzle them occasionally. Put your head on their knee and roll your eyes at them. Trust me, it never fails.

- Never refuse a cuddle… unless it's from a cat lover.

Take pride in your work. The longer the walk, the greater the pleasure.

- Look out for those that love you.
- Get yourself a pink squeaky ball. Squeak it loudly and often until someone shouts at you. It's always good for a laugh.
- Never go to bed on an argument or your master's bed. But definitely never on an argument.
- Start each day with enthusiasm but don't expect others to join in.
- Take pride in your work. The longer the walk, the greater the pleasure.
- Lead the way.

Chapter 51:

I owe you one

Of course, Abbot's not the only one who's helped me along the way. Many people have played key roles in keeping me safe, sane, motivated and hopeful. I owe them my life. I want to mention them here, before this book reaches its end. That may be unusual, but then I'm an unusual guy, so you'll just have to come to terms with that... I don't want these thanks tucked out of sight, as if these people are just an afterthought. To me that would suggest these people were of lesser importance, when in fact they're very important indeed. These people are often, if not always, in my thoughts.

At the very top of any list must come Denise. She waited a long time for me to come back to my senses while I ran, lied, hid and generally behaved like an idiot. She often believed more in me than I did in myself and she was the one constant throughout my years of turmoil. When many things fell by the wayside – sight, sense, friends, possessions and often hope – Denise remained constant, always forgiving, resilient and patient. Her love was often the only thing that stood between me and oblivion. I know my behaviour hurt her deeply and I'm very ashamed – but I appreciate what she did enormously. She always remained my best friend. When she said 'for better or for worse' some 21 years ago, she didn't know there'd be so much of the 'worse'. Nevertheless, she kept faith with me and I love her more today than ever before. The last six years have been the happiest we've known and I'm deeply sorry I didn't make this happen sooner.

The next one to thank is Abbot himself. Thanks to him I am now in a chapter of my life that is far happier than anything I could have imagined and much more than I deserve. He's a wonderful guide, a great protector and, most of all, my best mate.

For a guide dog and owner partnership to really work, the owner must be in love with his dog so it's just as well I am... I was from the moment I met him. When there have been problems in Abbot's work it's been our joint friendship and commitment which has carried us through. We behave like mates, looking out for each other as mates should. And not only do we work together, we also play together, a fact which may well be the secret to our successful partnership.

The other person who I must include in my personal heroes and heroines is my gran. Of all the people who've had any influence over my life in all its 48 years, of all the people I admire, Gran would always be at the top of any list. If there is any good in me at all, anything of grace or kindness, then it comes from her. She was a true woman of faith, a real socialist, with deeply held values and a passionate supporter of any and every person less fortunate than herself. (If you were to park your car on the pavement outside my gran's house you would get the sharp end of her tongue!) She taught me everything of any merit or value and she walks with me and Abbot every day. I feel her love in so many ways and hear her voice constantly, encouraging me, guiding me on and keeping me safe from harm. I miss her more than ever. My one regret is that she never got to meet Abbot.

I feel her love in so many ways...

My experience of sight impairment has taught me a great deal about loss but nothing in life prepared me for the loss of my gran. Years have now passed but my sense of loss is no less acute. She's in my heart always. (Bless you, Gran. I love you and miss you more than I can say. Your love is a beacon that lights all the shadows of my life. On those dark days when life seems just too difficult I can hear you whispering words of encouragement.) Actually, until Gran died I'd never faced the idea of being a grown-up. I had never had to. She would always clear up my mess, defend me even when I knew I was wrong and shelter me from reality. Losing her, whilst very sad, was her way of making me grow up. I suspect that if Gran were still here I may not have faced up to any of this at all. She knew I could do this long before I did. She told me so on her death bed.

She knew I could do this long before I did.

I'd also like to mention a few other key people...

- Thank you to Sue from Guide Dogs, the person who was responsible for the truly inspired matching of me with Abbot. Abbot's personality totally mirrors my own and I could not have had a dog that was better suited to my character. Sue was the poor lady who had to broach the subject of long cane training with me and she quite unjustly suffered all the anger I'd been saving up for years. I'm deeply ashamed of the way I behaved towards her that day. Much to Sue's amusement, though, I did complete my long cane training a couple of years ago. Her perseverance was obviously worth it.

- I want to thank Lynne my trainer, who took the time and trouble to find out my particular needs and adapted my training accordingly. Her patience and kindness are things I will never forget even though her arched eyebrow still fills me with dread. God bless you, Lynne. Denise, Abbott and I are forever in your debt.
- A heartfelt thank you to all the members of Guide Dogs and especially to my fellow branch members locally. They put up with me in the early days of volunteering – during my first year of having Abbot – and I'm so glad I did start campaigning then, because it's at the beginning when someone is enthusiastic that things like that should start. Since then we've made some progress with our campaigns, raised quite a bit of money and had a lot of fun along the way.
- A big thank you, too to Jan and Mick, Abbot's puppy walkers. Thank you for having the courage to let Abbot go. I know you must miss him so much.
- I also want to thank my oldest mate, George Adams. He's always stood by me and kept faith even when my behaviour was at its worst. He's never critical and is always patient and kind. He's a true gentleman, who strives to see the good in everyone. He's also a great musician and has featured in just about every band I've been in. Just this last month we've dusted off our instruments and formed a new band. I love him dearly.
- Then there's Dave Newton. Dave is a really positive influence. He's almost always up for a new project. We met through recording music and we've now made a couple of films. Dave has joined me and George in our latest band and played at many a Guide Dogs event. He's taken the

cause of sight impairment to heart and is now a passionate and eloquent advocate. Above all, he's my mate: we share the odd beer, we debate philosophy, politics and religion and whenever I need a fix of humour Dave can be relied upon to come up with the goods.

- A big thank you to David and Brenda, who have put up with all my ranting and raving over the years and been a great source of encouragement, as well as great providers of coffee and biscuits. I am particularly grateful to Brenda for her help with the first draft of this book and I enjoyed all our arguments over what I should include! Her skills were invaluable to me.
- I also want to thank Allan Taylor. As I've explained, all my adult life his music has guided, comforted, encouraged and soothed me. His music has led me to explore the work of other musicians and, more than anything, it's given me something to cling to at times when I was sailing very close to the edge. In recent years our friendship has grown and he's performed in several concerts for Guide Dogs. Allan wrote the song 'Good Friends' for the film *The Road Ahead* and the lyrics say more than I could articulate myself about the bond between guide dog and owner. Allan you really are a good friend.
- Finally, I would like to thank my family for sticking by me. In recent years we've grown closer again. In the past I caused them a great deal of hurt and I thank God that we've had the chance to be reconciled. I love them more than ever... so, Mum and Dad, here's to the future.

I'd like to thank my family for sticking by me...

Chapter 52:

My guardian angel

Seven years after registering as sight impaired I now feel like a different person. I have a new business, a new home, new freedoms and I've returned to many old interests that I'd abandoned because of my sight loss. I have spoken about how I used to regard sight impairment as a stigma, a label that carried with it a badge, which I felt unable to wear. That day back in the hospital I decided that if I must wear such a badge I would wear it whole-heartedly and with pride. I'm now a fully committed, card-carrying blindy.

All of this is thanks to Abbot. I owe him everything. I can't begin to tell you how much life has changed and how much better it is now. I look back on my old life and it's almost as if it belonged to another person.

Nevertheless, I have to admit that my sight impairment has left some scars that not even Abbot has been able to heal. On these pages I'm sure you've noticed some bitterness. I wasted too many years – from that day in 1987 when I was forced to give up my 'proper job' until almost ten years later – simply running away from being a blindy, a thing that scared me to the core.

Disappearing as I used to do for days on end and drinking myself silly was never a solution. As well as having my problems to face, I'd even have new ones because while I was in hiding I'd feel terrified that Denise would leave me not only because of my blindness or my unemployment, but also because of my latest disappearing act. If only I'd faced up to the truth sooner!

As I've already explained, my running and denial didn't just hurt Denise (although that was bad enough) – it hurt so many other people too. I didn't just quietly scuttle away on my own with my anger, I would mouth off to anyone who got in the way and I didn't care who got caught in the crossfire. I feel deeply ashamed of the way I behaved. Some of the people from those times were eventually very supportive and were just pleased to see me get my act together in the end. But some of them couldn't seem to move on because they were so hurt by my behaviour. I deeply regret this and I miss them terribly. I wish more than anything that I could make things right with these people. I've held too many grudges myself against people who've hurt me and in the end these grudges have only served to disable me further. Who needs that? I know only too well, though, how hard it is to let go of old hurts. If you're reading this and you're one of the many people who holds a grudge against me, I hope you will contact me. I want to make amends because at last the running has stopped.

OK, OK, I'll admit there are still odd days when I want to get the hell away and drink myself into oblivion so as to numb the anger. It's as I said earlier: I'm a recovering addict and I have to take each day at a time. On angry days I still go out looking for someone I can vent my spleen on. People who know me would never refer to me as laid-back but Abbot has helped me to become a person who is much more at ease with himself.

I had always believed that to be open and honest about my sight loss would place me in far too vulnerable a position: a position where I would be at the mercy of those around me. But Abbot has filled me with a strength that I could never have imagined. I now know that I was much more vulnerable in my former life than I could ever be now. What's so amazing is that the very thing I feared so much really isn't so scary after all, now that I'm here and facing it. I even like the way things are now! My biggest regret is that I didn't wake up to the idea of a guide dog sooner. When I look back on all those years without a dog I can only shake my head and wonder.

Who knows what the future holds on the 'road ahead'? I'm still afraid of the day when I will wake up and never see anything again. I know that one day the sight just won't return again... and yes, I admit it, that still really scares me. I also know that in the near future the old boy will have to hang up his harness and I know we'll both find that difficult... We're already struggling to come to terms with the decision but we're facing it together and getting through it, as we have done with so many issues, so many times already. He deserves a long, happy retirement and I intend to see he that gets it.

Eventually a new guide dog will come along and no doubt I'll fall in love with him or her too. (In case you're wondering, guide dogs do come in both sexes, but they're always neutered. We don't want them chasing other dogs down the street!) Even when a new dog comes along, I know that no one is going to replace Abbot. Abbot was the first and has been so much more than just a guide dog. He's the one that helped me adjust to being sight impaired – a true blindy. He's given me a belief in myself which the next dog will not have to do. Abbot is the one and only. He gave me back my life and he did that with so much love and grace that whenever I think of him I'll always smile. I'll be in his debt for eternity.

Oh, yes. And there will eventually come a day when Abbot will no longer be with us. I know that all those who love him will be heartbroken. However, he is like a guardian angel. I know I'll always feel his presence close by. And then one day I'll arrive at heaven's gate and St Peter will want to know why he should let me in. I will have to admit that I don't deserve it. He'll say: 'I'm sorry, you've been a lair and a cheat.' And he'll be right. 'You've been a drunk,' he'll add. True. 'You've been bitter and bad-tempered.' True again. 'You've been unfair to the people of Sunderland.' Ah, yes, I'll admit it. 'I'm sorry,' St Peter will go on, brisk and business-like. 'You're in the wrong place.' Then Abbot will pop his head round the gate and say, 'It's OK, Pete. He's with me.' I told you there was a certain kudos in hanging around with Abbot.

There's only one word left to say – a word I learned from Abbot: 'Forward!' I was just about to turn off my computer for the final time and bring this story to a close but Abbot's here and he's just pointed something out to me. As this book has perhaps shown you, change is painful, whatever change it is that you personally are going through. (People who've gradually lost some or all of their sight know that only too well.) You can either allow yourself to be consumed by the process of change or you can move forward. This is not an easy lesson to learn, but if you don't learn it, it'll kill you.

You can either allow yourself to be consumed by the process of change or you can move forward.

It's Abbot's duty to give you a parting blessing in the true monastic tradition...

Beyond that, since Abbot is abbot of this little community (me, you and anyone else who happens to be reading this book), it's his duty to give you a parting blessing in the true monastic tradition:

May your bowl always be full

May your walks be long and happy

May there always be space in front of the fire

May there always be someone to hold your paw

In return you must lead gently, guide true.
   And remember: forward, always forward.

Remember: forward, always forward.

Postscript:

Hope for the future?

If you are one of the 40 million people worldwide, who (according to WHO statistics) are blind, or if you have a loved one who is sight impaired, I wonder how you feel now, having read this book? Are you perhaps wondering if there is hope for people who are experiencing some of the things I've described?

Of course, there is always hope in life. Nevertheless, we must always remain realistic, even if we sometimes feel so desperate that a flimsy hope is all we can cling to. But what does 'realistic' mean in practice? Does it mean limiting our thinking to our old 'twin-set-and-pearlies' preconceptions? Fortunately, living in modern Britain with a sight impairment does not mean becoming a social outcast. Although there's still a long way to go, there are already bumpy bits of pavement at every pedestrian crossing, there are markings in Braille on lifts and the law is developing so as to protect the interests of people with a sight impairment. The government already has a scheme to provide cleaning or cooking support for those who need it and grants are available to provide assistive technology (such as speech recognition software) for people who regularly use computers. There are numerous private companies offering services or products and, of course, charitable organisations (such as the RNIB and Guide Dogs) are constantly campaigning for any gaps to be filled in. Besides all that, did you know it's even possible now to get electronic canes which beep? And guide dogs are already being trained up for teenagers.

Some people, like me, are trying to take advantage of everything available. And it's not only in the UK that things are going on. Did you know that there's at least one blind person in the world who has become a world-famous mountaineer? He's also training other sight impaired people to climb. His name is Erik Weihenmayer and he's written a book called *Touch The Top Of The World* (Plume 2002).

Erik even believes that his disability has given him an advantage... which explains why his next book was called *The Adversity Advantage* (Fireside Books 2008). Even if you can't see yourself, or your loved one, following his example and climbing up the nearest mountain, you could perhaps be open-minded enough to check out what is possible on level ground. Denial and depression are all very well, but practical action are easier to live with.

For those who might be newly experiencing sight loss, the best first point of contact for all information, be it social care, mobility, benefit advice, emotional support, assistive technologies, rehabilitation issues or any other matter, must be the RNIB Helpline on 03 123 9999. Of course, there's also a website: www.rnib.co.uk.

At the RNIB website you will find information about all kinds of eye conditions which result in sight impairment. You can also get information from:
- www.fightingblindness.ie/eyeconditions
- www.nystagmus.co.uk

To obtain information on rights, employment and other such issues go to:
- www.actionforblindpeople.org.uk or
- www.henshaws.org.uk — if you live in the North

For me, setting up my business has given me a lifestyle that accommodates my sight impairment. Other types of employment would have been problematic. If you think this may be a way forward for you or your loved one, contact the BBACT (The Blind Business Association Charitable Trust) on 0845 0450696 or log onto their website at www.bbact.org.uk. As well as offering business advice and support, they operate a grant scheme and can put you in touch with other sight impaired entrepreneurs.

If you are looking for help with assistive technology I would recommend you contact Aspire Consultancy (www.aspire-consultancy.co.uk) or call 01904 762788.

If you would like to find out about getting either a symbolic or a long cane and finding training to use this, contact Guide Dogs or the RNIB (details as before).

Obviously as Abbot's proud owner I can't recommend the merits of guide dog ownership highly enough. If you would like to explore the possibility of guide dog ownership further or if you would like to know more about the many other services provided by Guide Dogs, go to www.guidedogs.org.uk.

If you are struggling to find reading material in your preferred format then go to the RNIB National Library Service. (The full website address is: www.rnib.org.uk/xpedio/groups/public/documents/publicwebsite/public_libinfoser.hcsp.) This is the largest specialist library in the UK and has over 40,000 alternative format books.

For information about sight loss,
the best first point of contact is the RNIB.

If you need material transcribed, contact AIRS—a service available to all in the UK.

If you need written material transcribed into other formats such as Braille, moon, large print or audio material contact AIRS by phoning 0191 433 8450 or logging onto their website at www.airs.org.uk. Incidentally, although they are part of Gateshead council, they will provide services to anyone in the UK for a small charge.

If you need specially designed products of any kind try:
- www.cobolt.co.uk
- www.talkingbooks.co.uk
- www.calibre.org.uk
- www.cpod.info

If you want to keep up to date with all the latest sight impairment news then listen to In Touch on BBC Radio 4.

If something comes up and you need to find out about the law as it affects everybody, check out:
- www.direct.gov.uk/en/DisabledPeople/RightsAndObligations and
- www.dwp.gov.uk/employers/dda

Last but not least, if you'd like to find out about my films or the services my own company offers (for building or website audits, amongst other things) log onto www.roadahead.tv or phone 07530 631216. You may be able to improve your own or your loved one's situation by making other people more aware of what sight impairment really means. (I hope this book may help too!)

Beyond all these practical steps you can take, I would encourage you to stay in touch with your GP, consultant or ophthalmologist. Research into surgical and other medical technologies is continuing and surprising treatments may be available to people with certain kinds of sight impairment... now or at some point in the future.

Over the past century many researchers have looked for effective ways of helping people recover their eyesight, even if only partially. According to Milena Vurro, a researcher into visual neuroscience and visual prostheses at Newcastle University, one of the most important research discoveries over the past few decades was made in 1968 by G Brindley. He discovered that it was possible to make blind people perceive a spot of light (called a 'phosphene') by electrically stimulating parts of the visual pathway. Later research showed that stimulating the neural tissue at various points in the visual system using an implanted neural stimulator also caused people to perceive a distorted version of the same pattern. Several groups of researchers are now developing this form of treatment (called visual prosthesis), with different researchers focusing on stimulating different parts of the visual pathway – either the retina, the optic nerve, or the cerebral cortex, since stimulating each of these seems to be helpful with different types of visual disease.

Different researchers are focusing on different parts of the visual pathway to help with different types of disease.

For example with retinitis pigmentosa and macular degeneration (which only affect light receptors), the still functional layer of neurons in the retina can sometimes be successfully stimulated. Retinal prosthesis – as it is called – can take two forms. In the case of 'epi-retinal' prosthesis the sight impaired person wears an external camera attached to a pair of glasses, a mini-computer and a transmitter, while an electronic stimulator is attached to his or her retinas. In the case of 'sub-retinal' prosthesis (which was first tried in the year 2000), so-called microphotodiodes are attached to the back of the retinas. These devices enable the eyes to receive light as each photodiode acts as a photoreceptor.

Bear with me... I'm not trying to blind you with science! It just might be helpful to know about research going on.

Other amazing things can be tried for certain people. If the optimal nerve has become inflamed or damaged, optical nerve prostheses or cortical implants may be helpful (the latter involving an implant into the brain). Both these approaches also involve the use of a camera, a portable processor and a transmitter (as with epi-retinal prostheses). For people with cataracts, laser surgery may be able to remove them, and the success rate is fairly high.

In the case of any kind of surgery there are obviously high risks. A lot of research still needs to be conducted so as to determine the long-term effectiveness of visual prosthesis in particular and we need to remember that only a small number of people have tried it so far. All kinds of problems need to be resolved before it can become a practical reality for the severely sight impaired: power supplies need to be refined, better bio-materials need to be found which are compatible with neuro-biological tissue, packaging needs to be developed so that equipment will remain adequately protected until it is used and surgical techniques need to be improved so as to minimise the current high risk of infection and ensure that implants remain correctly positioned long term.

Given the risks, a person who has a sight impairment may prefer to consider using a dog or a traditional cane! It's nice to know, though, that research is continuing in this area because someday soon it may well mean that many people are able to benefit. In the future, the sight impaired who dare to try out these new technologies may find it easier to get around, recognise objects or people's faces and they may eventually even be able to read again, with the help of these visual prostheses.

Until that time, with the help of this book, I hope that you or your loved ones — or the people you know who are sight impaired — will take constructive steps to build a better future with the services and equipment that are available in your geographical area.

As with other problems in life, when we or our loved ones (or our clients!) experience sight impairment we should not give up all hope but instead look for different kinds of solutions. They are there for the finding if only we will look...

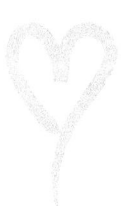

QUICK REFERENCE CONTACT LIST

For immediate pointers and support:
- www.rnib.co.uk
  Tel: 03 123 9999

For info on specific eyesight problems:
- www.rnib.co.uk
  Tel: 03 123 9999
- www.fightingblindness.ie/eyeconditions

For info on rights, work and the law:
- www.actionforblindpeople.org.uk
- www.henshaws.org.uk
  (in the North of England)
- www.direct.gov.uk/en/DisabledPeople/RightsAndObligations
- www.dwp.gov.uk/employers/dda

For info to set up your own business:
- www.bbact.org.uk
  Tel: 0845 0450696

For a building or website audit + films:
- www.roadahead.tv
  Tel: 07530 631216

For assistive technology:
- www.aspire-consultancy.co.uk
  Tel: 01904 762788

To get a cane and local training:
- www.rnib.co.uk
- www.aidmobility.co.uk
- www.guidedogs.org.uk

To find out about getting a guide dog:
- www.guidedogs.org.uk
  Tel: 0118 983 5555

To get hold of helpful products:
- www.cobolt.co.uk
- www.talkingbooks.co.uk
- www.calibre.org.uk
- www.cpod.info

To get more copies of this book:
- www.freshheartpublishing.co.uk

Do you have a story to share?

Do you live with someone who's sight impaired? Are you having problems with your own eyesight? Would you like to share your experiences with a view to helping other people? Your story could be posted on the Fresh Heart website—or perhaps it could also appear in a future book!

If you would like to share your personal experiences of sight impairment or life alongside someone who is sight impaired, please log onto the Fresh Heart Publishing website at www.freshheartpublishing.co.uk and click on 'Share Your Experience'. Alternatively, write to the following address:

'Share Your Experience'
Fresh Heart Publishing
PO Box 225
Chester le Street
DH3 9BQ

We'd love to hear from you!

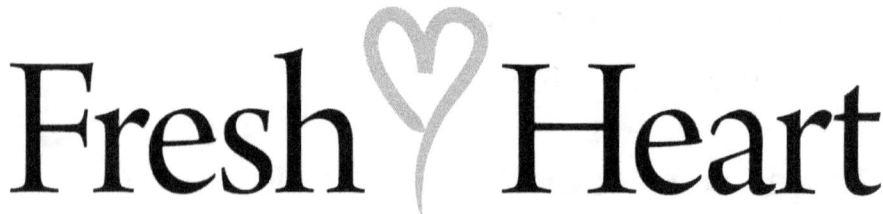

www.freshheartpublishing.co.uk

Want more copies of this book by post?

Photocopy this form, fill it in – obviously! – and send it, along with your cheque for the appropriate amount, to:

Fresh Heart Publishing, PO Box 225, Chester le Street, DH3 9BQ, United Kingdom

I would like _____ copies of *Stepping Into The Dark* [paperback edition] ISBN 978 1 906619 17 6 (£15 each)
Note: This is a discount price. The RRP for the books is £18.

I enclose a UK bank cheque payable to 'Fresh Heart' for £ _____. P&P is free for any number of books.
[Prices only for the UK. Other rates available on request.]

NAME: _____

ADDRESS:
_____
_____
_____

POSTCODE: _____

Email: _____

Telephone: _____

Send a cheque, not cash. Please allow 28 days for delivery. You can also place orders at www.freshheartpublishing.co.uk and get more info there about other Fresh Heart books.

For updates on prices, which may be subject to change, email sales@freshheartpublishing.co.uk or write to the address above.

Who is David Lucas?

Born and bred in Jarrow in the North East, David Lucas has had problems with his eyesight all his life. However, after starting off like most other people—in normal schools and jobs and doing the usual very ordinary things that people do—he's gradually become more and more sight impaired. Now, at the age of 49, he is officially registered 'severely sight impaired'.

Despite a harrowing emotional journey, David has at last come to terms with his sight impairment and discovered new ways of enjoying life. In this book he shares his story. He hopes that through reading about his difficulties (which he knows all too many people experience) people who come into contact with the sight impaired will gain a better understanding of sight impairment and all that it implies in terms of daily living.

David now works as an access auditor and low vision awareness trainer. He is also a committed campaigner for the rights of sight impaired people, working particularly with the charity Guide Dogs for the Blind as an adviser and fundraiser. Of course—given David's enduring love of music—he also still plays the guitar whenever he has time.

He still lives in Jarrow, with his wife Denise and their guide dog Abbot. While David claims to have come to terms with his sight impairment, he does still feel inclined to call himself the world's most reluctant blind man.

> He does still feel inclined to call himself the world's most reluctant blind man...

... but Dave has at last come to terms with his sight impairment.

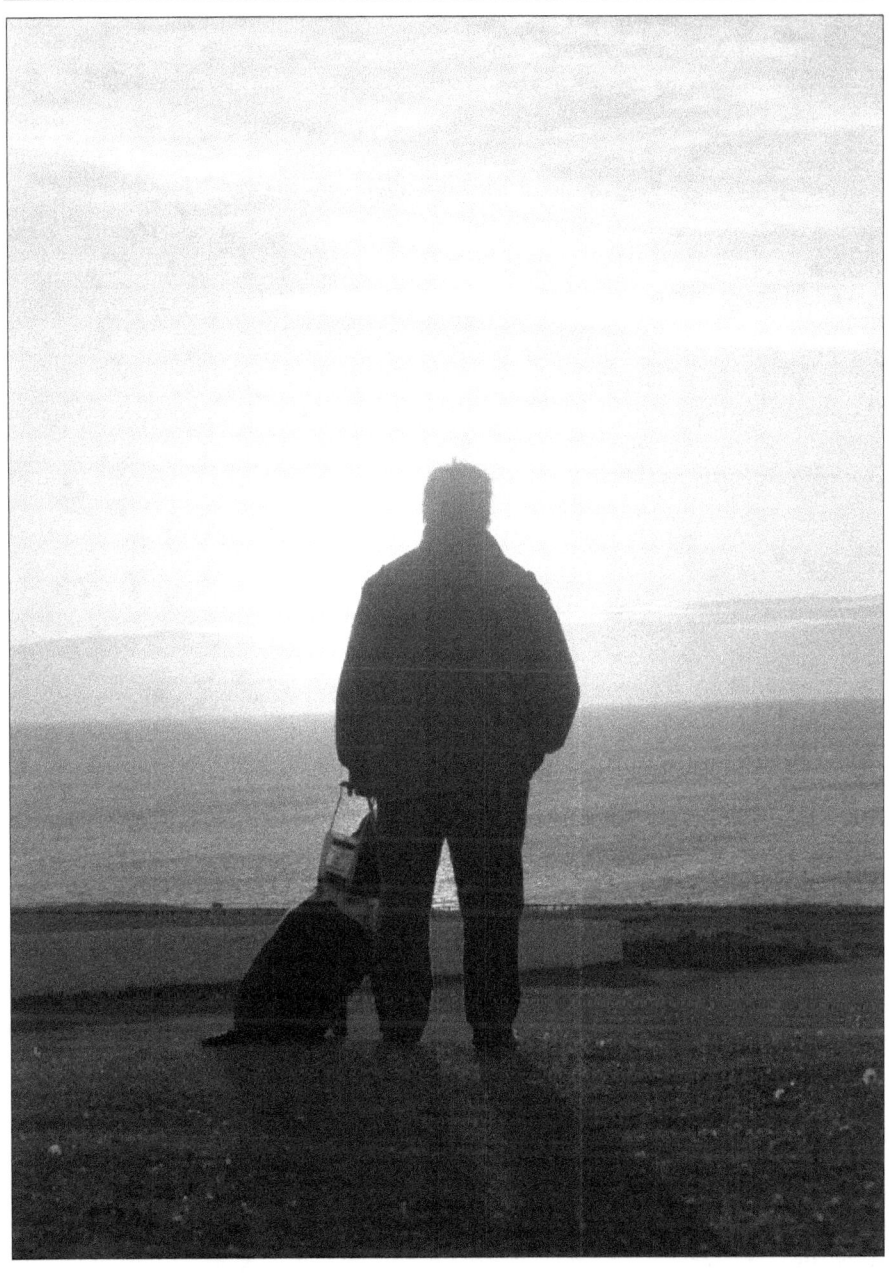

Photo of Dave and Abbot by Doug Blake

www.ingramcontent.com/pod-product-compliance
Lightning Source LLC
Chambersburg PA
CBHW062026220426
43662CB00010B/1485